the baby bump

twins and triplets edition

100s of secrets for those
9 long months with
multiples on board

Carley Roney

and the editors of TheBump.com

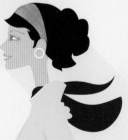

CHRONICLE BOOKS

SAN FRANCISCO

Page 176 constitutes a continuation of the
copyright page.

Library of Congress Cataloging-in-Publication
Data available.
ISBN 978-1-4521-0665-6

Manufactured in China

Design by Liza Aelion, Kelly Crook, Dawn Camner
Design assistance by Lydia Ortiz
Cover photo:
    Thinkstock
Cover illustration by
    LULU*/CWC International, Inc.
Back cover by Davies+Starr

The ideas, procedures, and suggestions contained in this
book are not intended as health care or other professional
advice, diagnosis, or a substitute for consulting with your
health care professional. Every baby is different and circumstances vary, so you should consult your own physician and use
your own common sense. The author and publisher offer no
warranties or guarantees, expressed or implied, in the com-
pleteness or advisability of the information contained in this
book for your particular situation, and disclaim any liability
arising from its use.

10 9 8 7 6 5 4 3 2 1

Chronicle Books LLC
680 Second Street
San Francisco, CA 94107
www.chroniclebooks.com

Contents

introduction

Double, triple, quadruple congrats! You're having twins—or more! With any pregnancy (especially the first), there are so many new things to think about, from what you can (and can't) eat to all that crazy stuff happening to your body. (Seriously, did anyone tell you your boobs would start looking bluish and your gums would bleed like this?)

But for moms-to-be of multiples, there are even more questions that your singleton-pregnancy pals won't ever have to think about: Can your babies kick each other? (No, that amniotic fluid is pretty tough.) What's a mixed delivery?(Just what it sounds like: one vaginal; one cesarean. They're not super-common, and if you're having multiples, you're pretty much guaranteed a c-section.) Will they grow at the same rate? (Probably not exactly but pretty close.) What are the chances they'll be identical? (Fraternal twins are far more common.) How come the doctor heard only one heartbeat? (Sometimes one baby will be behind another and muffle out the sound.) The list goes on and on, and don't worry—the answers on these pages go into a lot more depth. We'll give you the lowdown on everything mamas-to-be are wondering—and even those first few weeks when you bring babies home. Caring for one is tough enough, but once you add more, it can get pretty hairy if you don't have help.

And if you have more questions or just want to chat with other moms of multiples, go to TheBump.com/multiples. There are experts, message boards, and loads more info.

You're in for a crazy, thrilling, amazing time. And there are, oh, at least 1,000 things to figure out before your babies arrive. It's a good thing you have those 30-plus weeks to get ready. So get reading, but don't forget to enjoy the journey, too. There's nothing in the world like being pregnant. Having a baby (or two or three at once) rocks your world, but in a really good way.

week-by-week fetal development

week 5 →
Your babies are starting to form major organs, like the heart, kidneys, liver, and stomach, the nervous, circulatory, and digestive systems.

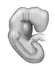

week 6 —
As blood starts to circulate, babies are starting to develop eyes, ears, a nose, cheeks, and a chin.

week 7 →
With joints starting to form, babies are developing arms and legs.

mom at 1 week

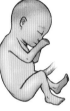

week 24 —
As fat starts to pack on, skin is becoming more opaque and, thanks to the formation of small capillaries, it's taking on a pink glow.

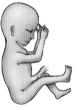

week 22 ←
Settling into sleep cycles, babies are sleeping 12 to 14 hours a day.

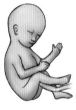

week 20 —
Each day, babies are gulping down several ounces of amniotic fluid for nutrition and to practice swallowing—and those taste buds actually work.

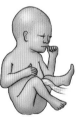

week 26 →
Babies are getting their immune system ready for life outside the womb by soaking up antibodies.

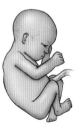

week 28 —
Their skin is still pretty wrinkly (one by-product of living in amniotic fluid) but will smooth out as fat continues to deposit.

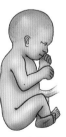

week 31 →
Your babies are going through major brain and nerve development. Their irises now react to light, and all five senses work.

week 8
Continuing to straighten in the trunk, babies can move those little arms, legs, and (slightly webbed) fingers and toes.

week 9 →
The little embryos are now officially fetuses, and a Doppler ultrasound device may be able to pick up the beating heart.

week 10
Arm joints are working as bones and cartilage are forming, and vital organs are starting to function.

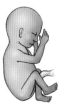

week 18 ←
Babies have become amazingly mobile as they yawn, hiccup, roll, twist, kick, punch, suck, and swallow.

week 16
Tiny bones are forming in their ears and eyebrows, and lashes and hair are starting to fill in.

week 13
While the intestines move from the umbilical cord to their tummies, babies are developing teeth and vocal cords.

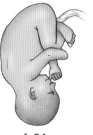

week 34
Babies can recognize and react to simple songs and may even remember them after birth. Less cute news: They now pee about a pint each day.

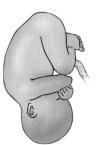

week 37 →
Your full-term (yay!) babies are gaining about half an ounce a day, and they're getting their first sticky poop (aka meconium) ready.

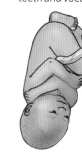

week 39
Babies' brains are still developing rapidly, and by now they're able to flex their limbs. Their nails also might start to extend past the fingertips.

mom at 40 weeks

chapter

did you say twins?

one

more good news! By the time the doctor tells you you're carrying multiples, you're probably well into your first trimester (that's why we start with week 8, not week 1). As you're getting over the shock of finding out there's not just one baby in there and probably feeling tired and overwhelmed and even struggling with morning sickness, you know you'll be turning the corner in just a few weeks. Wahoo! Plus, there's something huge to look forward to: This is the month when your OB will (probably) start listening to the babies' heartbeats at each visit—there's no cooler sound for a mama-to-be than the thump-thumping you're going to hear (don't be freaked out that it's fast; that's totally normal). So take the leftover nasties in stride and look forward to an increasing appetite, an increasing waistline, and (hopefully) a decreasing sense of having to throw up at any given moment.

your to-do list

- Schedule a CV screening
- Hear the heartbeats
- Eat for three (or more!)
- Buy a bigger bra

Connect with other mamas-to-be of multiples at TheBump.com/chat

what you're in for...

Weird—that sounds like a horse galloping.

I've got bluish veins showing up under the skin on my boobs.

I'M PEEING CONSTANTLY.

Another zit? And this one's on my back!

my boobs are getting huge!

I need TUMS. Now. (Hello, heartburn.)

OMG—there are *three* in there.

I'M CONSTANTLY HUNGRY.

twins!

I'm feeling cranky, tired, and nauseous.

on your mind...

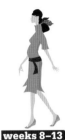

weeks 8–13

❚ I'm pregnant with multiples?

"Seriously. Twins? Any chance the doctor is wrong?"

If you've had a clinical exam (especially an initial ultrasound to see what's taking shape in there) that's confirmed the presence of more than one little guy, it's time to start celebrating, times two.

"What's the earliest my doctor can tell me if I'm having multiples?"

Even though multiples are formed between 4 and 10 days after conception (when more than one egg is fertilized or one embryo randomly splits), you probably won't learn that you're having twins until your first ultrasound appointment (around 10 weeks) when the tech yells, "It's twins!" As a newly minted mom of multiples, you'll experience many surprises, and this is only the first of many, so try not to fall off the table. You might be able to sense for yourself that you're having more than one baby, even before that first ultrasound. (One big hint: Your belly's growing faster than average.) Either way, you won't have to wait long before you'll know to start doubling up on baby supplies.

how big are they?

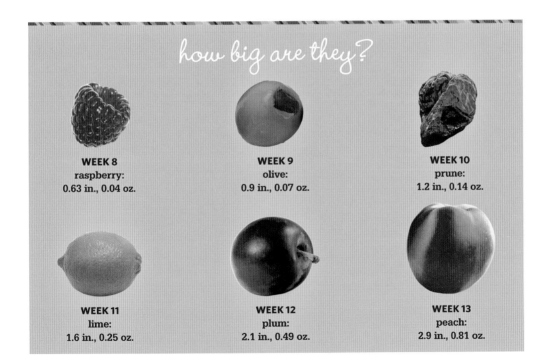

WEEK 8
raspberry:
0.63 in., 0.04 oz.

WEEK 9
olive:
0.9 in., 0.07 oz.

WEEK 10
prune:
1.2 in., 0.14 oz.

WEEK 11
lime:
1.6 in., 0.25 oz.

WEEK 12
plum:
2.1 in., 0.49 oz.

WEEK 13
peach:
2.9 in., 0.81 oz.

"So, what exactly were the chances of this, anyway?"

About 1 out of every 30 births (or about 3 percent) are twins. Once you go beyond twins to triplets or quadruplets, the chances drop significantly. About 148 of every 100,000 births (or 0.15 percent) are triplets or more. That said, your chances of pushing a double stroller go up if you're over 30, have a family history of fraternal twins, are African American, are obese or very tall, or were undergoing fertility treatments.

"So, having IVF made me more likely to have multiples?"

Just as in vitro fertilization ups your chances of getting pregnant, it also ups your chances of having more than just one baby. That's why the rise in popularity of fertility treatments (like IVF) has so strongly impacted the rise in multiple births over the last few decades. This tends to happen because more than one embryo is implanted in order to increase the chance of pregnancy, and multiple embryos potentially mean multiple babies! In fact, IVF babies are 20 times more likely to be multiples than naturally conceived babies. Some studies even say that close to half of the babies born thanks to IVF treatments are multiples.

"Now that I know I'm having twins, how likely are they to be fraternal versus identical twins?"

Let's backtrack here to the moment of conception. It was a hot summer night.

Okay, just kidding—we don't have to go that far back. Let's skip to the part where sperm meets egg and, voilà, you have a baby (you probably already knew that part). Now, if your body releases more than one egg, a separate sperm can fertilize each one and you'll be welcoming your fraternal (or, in fancy terms, dizygotic) twins. This is the most likely scenario—about two-thirds of all twins are fraternal. Each fraternal twin has his or her own placenta and amniotic sac. You can have two boys, two girls, or one of each, and in most cases they'll look no more alike than any other siblings, except that they happen to share the same birthday. Identical twins are much less common—about a third of all twin births. Their fancy name is monozygotic, or one egg. These guys are created when a fertilized egg splits very early in the pregnancy and develops into two separate fetuses with the same genetic material. They'll have the same eye color, hair color, and blood type.

"The doctor told me I'm having twins, but could there be even more in there?"

No medical device is 100 percent accurate all the time, so there's a chance that an ultrasound missed an extra sac and baby number 3 is playing hide-and-seek. But it's not very likely. Unfortunately, there is a possibility of something called vanishing twin syndrome, where one of the fetuses is miscarried and reabsorbed into the uterus. No one really knows what causes this and what, if anything, you can do to prevent it.

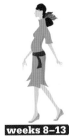

weeks 8–13

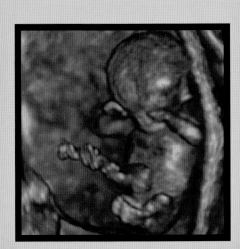

what babies are up to

- intestines develop more
- graduate from "embryo" to "fetus" at week 5
- arm and leg joints start working
- fingers and toes lose webbing
- vital organs begin to function
- bones and cartilage develop
- teeth and vocal cords form
- arms and feet start to take shape
- hair follicles, tooth buds, nail beds form

Editors note: We are showing you singleton sonograms throughout so you can really see the detail.

The danger is usually over by around week 12, so by then you can breathe a little easier.

"Do I need to find an OB who specializes in multiples? How can I find one?"
Not necessarily. A well-trained generalist (which, of course, we hope yours is!) can easily take good care of you if you're carrying twins and is a fine place to start. But you may need a little extra care. Since you're at a slightly higher risk for complications, your OB will likely consult with a maternal-fetal medicine specialist who has loads of experience dealing with twins, triplets, quads, quints (you get the idea). That means you may be sent to another office or specialist early on for your ultrasounds (all ultrasounds should be done by AIUM-certified centers), then possibly passed back to your general OB for your monthly check-ins and delivery. If you're expecting more than two, though, you're probably safest seeing a specialist from the get-go. Your doctor should be able to recommend a pro, but if you want to check out some names yourself, you can find a full listing on the Society for Maternal-Fetal Medicine website (www.smfm.org).

what's your due date?

There's no way to know for sure your delivery date. Here's how to get an idea: Simply find the first day of your last menstrual period (LMP) on this chart. Then look at the estimated date of delivery (EDD) directly below it.

LMP jan
1	2	3	4	5	6	7	8	9	10	11	12	13	14	15	16	17	18	19	20	21	22	23	24	25	26	27	28	29	30	31

EDD oct/nov
| 8 | 9 | 10 | 11 | 12 | 13 | 14 | 15 | 16 | 17 | 18 | 19 | 20 | 21 | 22 | 23 | 24 | 25 | 26 | 27 | 28 | 29 | 30 | 31 | 1 | 2 | 3 | 4 | 5 | 6 | 7 |

LMP feb
| 1 | 2 | 3 | 4 | 5 | 6 | 7 | 8 | 9 | 10 | 11 | 12 | 13 | 14 | 15 | 16 | 17 | 18 | 19 | 20 | 21 | 22 | 23 | 24 | 25 | 26 | 27 | 28 |

EDD nov/dec
| 8 | 9 | 10 | 11 | 12 | 13 | 14 | 15 | 16 | 17 | 18 | 19 | 20 | 21 | 22 | 23 | 24 | 25 | 26 | 27 | 28 | 29 | 30 | 1 | 2 | 3 | 4 | 5 |

LMP mar
| 1 | 2 | 3 | 4 | 5 | 6 | 7 | 8 | 9 | 10 | 11 | 12 | 13 | 14 | 15 | 16 | 17 | 18 | 19 | 20 | 21 | 22 | 23 | 24 | 25 | 26 | 27 | 28 | 29 | 30 | 31 |

EDD dec/jan
| 8 | 9 | 10 | 11 | 12 | 13 | 14 | 15 | 16 | 17 | 18 | 19 | 20 | 21 | 22 | 23 | 24 | 25 | 26 | 27 | 28 | 29 | 30 | 31 | 1 | 2 | 3 | 4 | 5 | 6 | 7 |

LMP apr
| 1 | 2 | 3 | 4 | 5 | 6 | 7 | 8 | 9 | 10 | 11 | 12 | 13 | 14 | 15 | 16 | 17 | 18 | 19 | 20 | 21 | 22 | 23 | 24 | 25 | 26 | 27 | 28 | 29 | 30 |

EDD jan/feb
| 8 | 9 | 10 | 11 | 12 | 13 | 14 | 15 | 16 | 17 | 18 | 19 | 20 | 21 | 22 | 23 | 24 | 25 | 26 | 27 | 28 | 29 | 30 | 31 | 1 | 2 | 3 | 4 | 5 | 6 |

LMP may
| 1 | 2 | 3 | 4 | 5 | 6 | 7 | 8 | 9 | 10 | 11 | 12 | 13 | 14 | 15 | 16 | 17 | 18 | 19 | 20 | 21 | 22 | 23 | 24 | 25 | 26 | 27 | 28 | 29 | 30 | 31 |

EDD feb/mar
| 8 | 9 | 10 | 11 | 12 | 13 | 14 | 15 | 16 | 17 | 18 | 19 | 20 | 21 | 22 | 23 | 24 | 25 | 26 | 27 | 28 | 1 | 2 | 3 | 4 | 5 | 6 | 7 | 8 | 9 | 10 |

LMP june
| 1 | 2 | 3 | 4 | 5 | 6 | 7 | 8 | 9 | 10 | 11 | 12 | 13 | 14 | 15 | 16 | 17 | 18 | 19 | 20 | 21 | 22 | 23 | 24 | 25 | 26 | 27 | 28 | 29 | 30 |

EDD mar/apr
| 8 | 9 | 10 | 11 | 12 | 13 | 14 | 15 | 16 | 17 | 18 | 19 | 20 | 21 | 22 | 23 | 24 | 25 | 26 | 27 | 28 | 29 | 30 | 31 | 1 | 2 | 3 | 4 | 5 | 6 |

LMP july
| 1 | 2 | 3 | 4 | 5 | 6 | 7 | 8 | 9 | 10 | 11 | 12 | 13 | 14 | 15 | 16 | 17 | 18 | 19 | 20 | 21 | 22 | 23 | 24 | 25 | 26 | 27 | 28 | 29 | 30 | 31 |

EDD apr/may
| 8 | 9 | 10 | 11 | 12 | 13 | 14 | 15 | 16 | 17 | 18 | 19 | 20 | 21 | 22 | 23 | 24 | 25 | 26 | 27 | 28 | 29 | 30 | 1 | 2 | 3 | 4 | 5 | 6 | 7 | 8 |

LMP aug
| 1 | 2 | 3 | 4 | 5 | 6 | 7 | 8 | 9 | 10 | 11 | 12 | 13 | 14 | 15 | 16 | 17 | 18 | 19 | 20 | 21 | 22 | 23 | 24 | 25 | 26 | 27 | 28 | 29 | 30 | 31 |

EDD may/june
| 8 | 9 | 10 | 11 | 12 | 13 | 14 | 15 | 16 | 17 | 18 | 19 | 20 | 21 | 22 | 23 | 24 | 25 | 26 | 27 | 28 | 29 | 30 | 31 | 1 | 2 | 3 | 4 | 5 | 6 | 7 |

LMP sep
| 1 | 2 | 3 | 4 | 5 | 6 | 7 | 8 | 9 | 10 | 11 | 12 | 13 | 14 | 15 | 16 | 17 | 18 | 19 | 20 | 21 | 22 | 23 | 24 | 25 | 26 | 27 | 28 | 29 | 30 |

EDD june/july
| 8 | 9 | 10 | 11 | 12 | 13 | 14 | 15 | 16 | 17 | 18 | 19 | 20 | 21 | 22 | 23 | 24 | 25 | 26 | 27 | 28 | 29 | 30 | 1 | 2 | 3 | 4 | 5 | 6 | 7 |

LMP oct
| 1 | 2 | 3 | 4 | 5 | 6 | 7 | 8 | 9 | 10 | 11 | 12 | 13 | 14 | 15 | 16 | 17 | 18 | 19 | 20 | 21 | 22 | 23 | 24 | 25 | 26 | 27 | 28 | 29 | 30 | 31 |

EDD july/aug
| 8 | 9 | 10 | 11 | 12 | 13 | 14 | 15 | 16 | 17 | 18 | 19 | 20 | 21 | 22 | 23 | 24 | 25 | 26 | 27 | 28 | 29 | 30 | 31 | 1 | 2 | 3 | 4 | 5 | 6 | 7 |

LMP nov
| 1 | 2 | 3 | 4 | 5 | 6 | 7 | 8 | 9 | 10 | 11 | 12 | 13 | 14 | 15 | 16 | 17 | 18 | 19 | 20 | 21 | 22 | 23 | 24 | 25 | 26 | 27 | 28 | 29 | 30 |

EDD aug/sep
| 8 | 9 | 10 | 11 | 12 | 13 | 14 | 15 | 16 | 17 | 18 | 19 | 20 | 21 | 22 | 23 | 24 | 25 | 26 | 27 | 28 | 29 | 30 | 31 | 1 | 2 | 3 | 4 | 5 | 6 |

LMP dec
| 1 | 2 | 3 | 4 | 5 | 6 | 7 | 8 | 9 | 10 | 11 | 12 | 13 | 14 | 15 | 16 | 17 | 18 | 19 | 20 | 21 | 22 | 23 | 24 | 25 | 26 | 27 | 28 | 29 | 30 | 31 |

EDD sep/oct
| 8 | 9 | 10 | 11 | 12 | 13 | 14 | 15 | 16 | 17 | 18 | 19 | 20 | 21 | 22 | 23 | 24 | 25 | 26 | 27 | 28 | 29 | 30 | 1 | 2 | 3 | 4 | 5 | 6 | 7 | 8 |

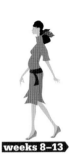

weeks 8–13

at the ob's office

"How often do I see the OB?"

You'll probably find yourself flipping through waiting room magazines far more often than some of your friends who are just carrying one baby. Your visits will depend largely on the number of babies you're carrying. If you're pregnant with nonidentical twins (aka dizygotic, meaning two of your eggs were fertilized by two of your partner's different sperm) you get a bit of a break in the appointment department. Once you've gone for your first trimester screening (typically between 11 and 14 weeks), you'll be back every month or so—at first for another set of screenings (15 to 20 weeks) and then for your anatomy scan (18 to 22 weeks). The monthly check-ins continue from then until your delivery day.

However, if your twins are identical (monozygotic) and share the same placenta or both the placenta and amniotic sac, you'll step it up a bit, hopping up on the OB's exam table once every two weeks. Same deal for triplets and beyond—about once every couple of weeks till D-day. Why the extra check-ins? For identical twins, who typically share a placenta, there's a higher risk that your babies may develop twin-to-twin transfusion syndrome, where one twin receives significantly more nutrition than his roommate. And because there's a significantly higher risk of preterm

multiples 101

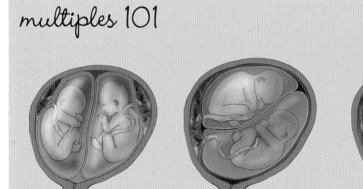

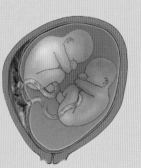

Dichorionic Diamniotic:
Fraternal or identical twins who have their own placenta and amniotic sac.

Monochorionic Diamniotic:
Identical twins who share the same placenta but have different amniotic sacs

Monochorionic Monoamniotic:
Identical twins who share the same placenta and amniotic sac

delivery from triplets and beyond, your doctor will likely want to stay on top of any potential changes happening inside.

"Will my checkups be different from my friends' who are carrying only one baby?"

In the beginning, there probably won't be too much difference between your pregnancy and those of ordinary folks who have only one passenger along for the ride. You will have more ultrasounds, though (see below for an exact rundown of how much more often). And as your belly (and everything else) gets bigger, your doctor may start to do some fetal monitoring around the 30-week mark. Don't stress—it's just another way for her to make sure everyone's getting all the nutrition they need.

"What exactly is going to happen at my first OB appointment?"

Your first trip usually includes a lot of poking and prodding. Expect to give a complete medical history and to have a full physical—pelvic exam, breast exam, urine test, pap smear, blood work—even if you recently had your annual GYN checkup. You'll also get lots of questions about your partner's family history, so try to bring him along (or all the answers you can dig up).

Here's the breakdown of what else to expect during that first appointment:

GENETIC TEST COUNSELING Your OB will talk about genetic testing and warning signs

to watch for. This is routine, so don't be alarmed.

GETTING A DUE DATE The OB will give you an estimated (now, we said *estimated!*) due date.

ULTRASOUND EXAM This is when your OB may be able to tell you that you are expecting more than one. In some cases, it may take a few more weeks, but if your OB can see more than one gestational sac or if there are two embryos (sometimes they share a gestational sac) on the monitor, you're carrying multiples! (Quick vocab lesson: Ultrasound is the name of the procedure; the sonogram is the image that's created.)

This is also the time when the doc will discuss risks, lifestyle changes, and the long list of no-nos for you. There are increased health concerns for mamas-to-be of multiples, so pay close attention and don't be shy about jumping in with your questions.

You and your OB will also work out a schedule for the rest of your appointments. It varies by doctor, but the typical time frame is one visit a month until 28 weeks, two visits a month until 32 weeks, and once a week after that until your babies are born.

"So, how often will I need to get ultrasounds?"

You can expect your OB to do an early ultrasound on your first office visit post-conception, just to make sure everything's okay. If you're transporting fraternal twins

"what questions do I need to ask my OB if I'm having multiples?"

• Should I see an MFM (maternal-fetal medicine specialist, perinatologist) during my pregnancy?

These MDs have received higher levels of training specifically for high-risk pregnancies and can help ensure you're being monitored appropriately.

• Does each baby have its own placenta and amniotic sac?

Babies who share a placenta and amniotic sac need to be watched closely to ensure they remain healthy in their shared space.

• Are my babies the same size?

Your babies should grow at about the same rate. If one's smaller than the other, this may be a sign of distress.

• Are the amniotic fluid levels balanced?

Excess amniotic fluids are also a potential sign of distress.

• What is my cervical length?

This is something that many doctors often overlook. A thinning or shortening cervix can be a telltale sign of a problematic pregnancy.

or triplets, you'll get your big anatomy scan between weeks 18 and 22. Prepare to settle in—because your OB will be looking at everything (heart, lungs, liver) times two (or more), the scan can take a good 45 minutes or more. After that, expect to get an in-the-womb look every four weeks, starting at about your 26th week. Why the frequent peeks? Your doctor is just making sure everyone is growing at the right rate and getting along (yes, they're learning to share and play nice even now). Special shout-out to moms of identical twins: Because there are more issues involved (these babies are sharing blood, fluids, placenta—all the good stuff), plan to be under the wand even more frequently. Your OB will likely be checking monthly growth scans, and also will be doing a fluid check by looking at your amniotic sac every two weeks to make sure everything is going well in the sac.

"How do I know if I'm Rh negative or Rh positive?"

At your first prenatal appointment, your OB will take blood for a long list of screenings. One of them will be to determine your blood type. You may already know if you're type A or O, but what's important during pregnancy is whether or not you're "positive" or "negative." Your OB will test your blood for Rh, a protein present in about 85 percent of the population. If you're Rh-negative and the father is Rh-positive, the fetus can inherit the Rh factor from the father. This makes the fetus Rh-positive too. Problems can arise when the fetus's blood has the Rh factor and the mother's blood does not. So, baby is "positive" but you are "negative." If this happens, it's possible for you to develop antibodies to your baby, in essence your body will think it's allergic to baby. To prevent any complications, you'll need injections of a medication called RhoGAM

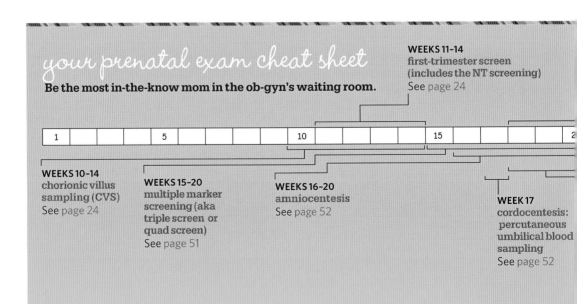

your prenatal exam cheat sheet
Be the most in-the-know mom in the ob-gyn's waiting room.

WEEKS 11–14
first-trimester screen
(includes the NT screening)
See page 24

| 1 | | | | 5 | | | | | 10 | | | | | 15 | | | | | 2 |

WEEKS 10–14
chorionic villus
sampling (CVS)
See page 24

WEEKS 15–20
multiple marker
screening (aka
triple screen or
quad screen)
See page 51

WEEKS 16–20
amniocentesis
See page 52

WEEK 17
cordocentesis:
percutaneous
umbilical blood
sampling
See page 52

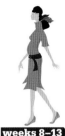

weeks 8–13

at 28 or 29 weeks and 72 hours before delivery to prevent problems.

"How would I know if I were having a miscarriage?"

It's normal to worry, but remember that most pregnancies end with healthy, happy babies. If you do experience a miscarriage, though, the first sign is usually vaginal bleeding. (There are other reasons for bleeding, too, so don't panic. Just call your OB.) Other signs include pelvic cramps, abdominal pain, and lower back pain.

"The doctor isn't seeing a dividing line between the twins. What does that mean?"

Some twins learn to share at a very young age. The majority of identical twins will share the same placenta but have separate amniotic sacs (monochorionic diamniotic), although a smaller percentage of identicals have their own of each one (dichorionic diamniotic). When there's sharing involved, there's a higher risk of complications, so you'll likely be getting some extra attention from your doctor, and will almost definitely be referred to a maternal-fetal medicine specialist. One serious potential complication is twin-to-twin transfusion syndrome, where one twin gets too much blood and nutrients while the other doesn't get enough. It's still a relatively rare occurrence, but if your twins are sharing a placenta, let's just say you'll become very familiar with the magazines in her waiting room.

"What does the heart rate mean?"

Your OB will likely listen for the heartbeats with a Doppler ultrasound around weeks 10 through 12. Anything between 110 and 160 beats per minute this early in your pregnancy is considered "normal" and healthy.

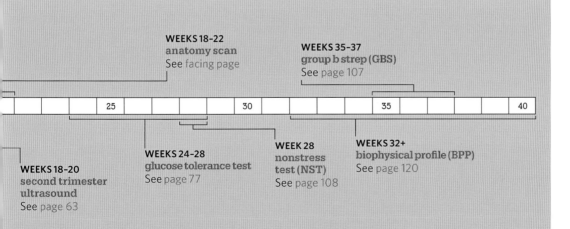

WEEKS 18-22
anatomy scan
See facing page

WEEKS 35-37
group b strep (GBS)
See page 107

25   30   35   40

WEEKS 24-28
glucose tolerance test
See page 77

WEEK 28
nonstress test (NST)
See page 108

WEEKS 32+
biophysical profile (BPP)
See page 120

WEEKS 18-20
second trimester ultrasound
See page 63

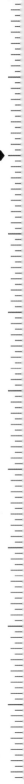

Although you may have heard your grandma claim that the heart rates can reveal your babies' genders, scientists say no way. In fact, the heart rate of each baby can change from moment to moment, depending on activity; if one of your babies is wiggling around, that can cause the heart to speed up a bit. (But if you want to play along for fun, the old wives' tale claims that girls' hearts beat faster.)

"What's an NT screening? I've heard of it but don't know if I need one."

The nuchal translucency (or NT) screening is a special ultrasound performed between weeks 11 and 14 (it's part of the first-trimester screen), so your doctor can check the volume of the clear, fluid-filled space in the back of each of your babies' growing necks. A high volume of fluid can be an early indicator of Down syndrome, trisomy 18, and other chromosomal abnormalities, as well as congenital heart defects.

This scan is often done in combination with a serum test to check certain hormone levels in your blood. (You might hear the full deal referred to as your "first-trimester screening.") This screening won't get you any definite answers—only an alert for potential risks. If the results are abnormal, your doctor will offer more tests, like a CVS (which is more accurate than the NT and done between weeks 10 and 14). The NT test is optional, which means that it's not one of the essential screenings performed during pregnancy.

"I'm going to have prenatal diagnostic testing done. How do I decide between CVS and an amnio?"

Both have benefits. CVS (chorionic villus sampling) is done earlier, anytime between 10 and 14 weeks, so it means putting an end to your worries sooner or, in a worst-case scenario, giving you more time to reflect on the results. The CVS test is a biopsy of the placenta (or placentas) in order to diagnose your babies with possible chromosomal disorders.

An amniocentesis cannot be performed until after week 15 of your pregnancy, because doctors typically wait until the babies develop and the chances of harming them decrease. The test involves inserting a needle into your bump to draw fluid from the sac (or sacs) that surround your little ones. The fluid is then analyzed for abnormalities. If you're at particular risk for neural tube defects (such as spina bifida), an amnio is the clear choice, because CVS won't detect these. An amnio, which is usually done between weeks 15 and 18, allows you to postpone making a decision (to test or not to test) until after you've seen the results of your second-trimester screenings.

"What's a chorionicity scan, and why do I need one?"

A chorionicity scan helps determine whether or not your babies are sharing a placenta. If you have a multiple pregnancy, you'll want to ask for a chorionicity scan to find this

"how much more do I need to eat?"

If you're expecting twins, guidelines say you should consume 300 extra calories per day in the first trimester, 680 in the second trimester, and 900 in the third. If you're carrying triplets, eat 450 extra calories in the first trimester, 1,020 in the second trimester, and 1,350 in the third. Keep in mind that the sources of the calories are even more important than the number you consume. Get 20 to 25 percent of your calories from protein, 45 to 50 percent of your calories from carbs (but stay away from white carbs—moms carrying multiples are at increased risk for gestational diabetes), and 30 percent of your calories from fats.

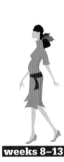

weeks 8–13

zinc
HOW MUCH 30 mg per day
WHY Zinc levels drop off during pregnancy, so make sure to supplement your diet with this essential nutrient that is linked to a lower risk of preterm delivery, low birth weight, and prolonged labor.
TRY Black-eyed peas are a great choice.

folic acid
HOW MUCH 600 µg a day
WHY Even before you get pregnant, you should start increasing this one. Doing so cuts your risk of birth defects.
TRY No midnight cravings for spinach or asparagus? Try an orange for 50 µg a pop.

calcium
HOW MUCH If you're expecting twins, get 1,500 mg a day, and get 2,000 mg a day if you're carrying triplets.
WHY It's extremely important to get enough calcium when pregnant. This essential nutrient can reduce the severity and lower the overall risk of preeclampsia, low birth weight, and preterm delivery.
TRY Some yogurt has 450 mg per cup, which is more than the calcium in a serving of milk!

magnesium
HOW MUCH 300 mg per day
WHY This decreases risk of premature labor and aids in developing your babies' nervous systems.
TRY Sprinkling some almonds on your cereal! Nuts are a great source, and a quarter cup of almonds has 98 mg of magnesium.

protein
HOW MUCH Calculate your nonpregnant protein needs (an average-size woman needs 70 g of protein a day) and add 25 g of protein per fetus.
WHY Your body needs a lot more protein now to help the fetuses grow and ensure that your babies' muscles develop properly.
TRY A lean-beef or chicken burger yields 30 g.

DHA
HOW MUCH There are no specific guidelines for how much DHA a mom of multiples should be getting each day, but some studies say you should be aiming for 600 mg per day.
WHY Higher levels of DHA in newborns correspond with higher birth weights. It's also associated with higher IQs, advanced motor skills, and fewer neurological problems later.
TRY A 4-oz. serving of salmon packs a punch, with 130 mg.

iron
HOW MUCH 30 mg per day
WHY Not enough can impair your babies' growth and increase the risk of hypertension, preterm delivery, and low birth weight.
TRY A bowl of fortified cereal at 10 mg, which provides more iron than a serving of beef.

vitamin D
HOW MUCH 25 µg per day
WHY It helps increase blood circulation in the placenta and aids in calcium absorption so that your babies will have improved bone mass.
TRY A fortified cup of orange juice, or go outside and get some sun for a few minutes every day, because this vitamin can be absorbed through sun exposure.

out early on, so you can determine if your babies are at risk for twin-to-twin transfusion syndrome. Babies who do share a placenta should be monitored extra-carefully for this condition to ensure that you have the healthiest pregnancy possible.

❚ in your head

"Why am I considered high risk, and what does that even mean?"

The fact of the matter is that you're more at risk for complications compared with someone whose uterus is housing just one baby right now, including both delivering before Junior is fully cooked (aka having a preemie) and developing some pregnancy-related health issues yourself (diabetes, high blood pressure, etc.). And the more babies you have on board, the higher the chance—albeit still a relatively small one—of something going wrong. So while it's important to make sure you're following all the healthy-pregnancy rules that you can (eat right, get lots of sleep, keep up those doctor's appointments), don't panic. It's under control.

"Are there different questions I need to ask my doctor if I conceived multiples naturally, versus through IVF?"

Yes. Multiples conceived through IVF (ICSI and assisted hatching) are usually fraternal and may not share the same placenta or amniotic sac, like identical twins do. Babies who share the same placenta

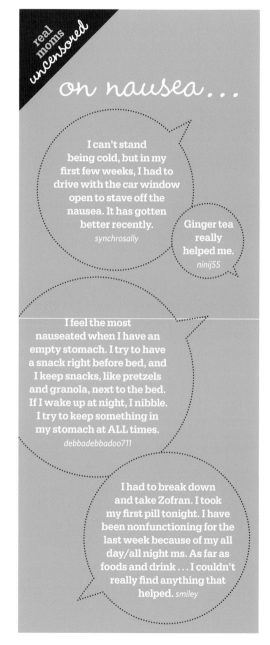

real moms uncensored

on nausea...

I can't stand being cold, but in my first few weeks, I had to drive with the car window open to stave off the nausea. It has gotten better recently. *synchrosally*

Ginger tea really helped me. *ninij55*

I feel the most nauseated when I have an empty stomach. I try to have a snack right before bed, and I keep snacks, like pretzels and granola, next to the bed. If I wake up at night, I nibble. I try to keep something in my stomach at ALL times. *debbadebbadoo711*

I had to break down and take Zofran. I took my first pill tonight. I have been nonfunctioning for the last week because of my all day/all night ms. As far as foods and drink... I couldn't really find anything that helped. *smiley*

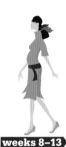

weeks 8–13

(monochorionic babies) have the highest risk of complications. Monochorionic gestations occur in two-thirds of identical twins and are at a higher risk for a rare but serious condition called twin-to-twin transfusion syndrome (TTTS), which happens when one of the babies is unable to get enough blood, while the other has too much. If your babies are monochorionic, you'll want to ask your doctor to monitor your pregnancy extraclosely, since TTTS is a condition that can be corrected with early detection.

"Is there a chance of having two sets of identical twins?"

While it's possible, having double twins (meaning two eggs split twice) is highly improbable. Identical twins count for just 0.4 percent of all births, or about 1 in 300. The chance of both of those eggs splitting twice is almost unheard of, although there's been at least one documented case. Note that almost two-thirds of twin births are considered "spontaneous" (natural) while the remaining third come through assisted reproduction technologies like IVF. In that field, doctors are working to get twin and triplet rates down by implanting fewer embryos and cutting back on growing the fertilized eggs to blastocysts before implanting them.

"What exactly is twin-to-twin transfusion syndrome?"

The medical definition of twin-totwin transfusion syndrome (TTTS) is an unbalanced blood flow between monochorionic (MC) fetuses. Monochorionic twins are twins who share the same placenta, which means they also share blood vessels that distribute blood flow between each baby. For reasons that are unknown, 10 to 15 percent of MC twin fetuses will develop an uneven flow of blood between the shared blood vessels, resulting in TTTS. The smaller twin (aka the "donor twin") doesn't receive enough blood, while the larger twin (aka the "recipient twin") becomes overloaded with too much blood. In an attempt to reduce its blood volume, the recipient twin will up the amount of urine it produces, which causes its bladder to grow large and too much amniotic fluid to surround it. At the same time, the donor twin will produce an unusually low amount of urine and the amniotic fluid around the twin will lessen or disappear altogether.

Over the course of a pregnancy, TTTS will cause one twin to overdevelop, while the other will suffer from underdevelopment. Left untreated, TTTS can result in the loss of one or both twins and present serious developmental issues for surviving babies.

If you're panicking while reading this, here's some good news: In a handful of centers throughout the United States, a breakthrough TTTS treatment is now available that can reverse the effects of the condition. The earlier a pregnancy undergoes TTTS treatment, the greater the potential is for saving each baby, so speak to your doctor immediately about your options if you've just been diagnosed or are looking to be checked out.

"What is vanishing twin syndrome? I'm having twins; is this something I should worry about?"
In some cases, one fetus in a multiple pregnancy will die in the womb and the fetal tissue will be condensed in its sac by the other twin, placenta, or mother, giving the appearance that the baby has literally disappeared. This is what we call vanishing

twin syndrome (VTS). VTS usually occurs in the first trimester, and rarely are real medical risks, to either the mom or the other twin, associated with it when it does happen this early on.

"How long should I wait before telling my family and friends I'm carrying twins?"
This one's totally up to you. Chances are, you'll know you're pregnant before you are made aware that you're expecting multiples, so do

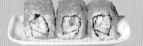

"what can I order at my favorite sushi restaurant?"

While lots of the menu is off-limits (since raw or seared fish can contain parasites and/or bacteria that can hurt your babies), there's still plenty to eat. Dig in!

	EAT
HOT APPETIZERS	edamame, shrimp shu mai, beef negimaki
SOUP	miso soup, udon or soba noodle soup
SALAD	field-greens salad, seaweed salad
SUSHI	eel-cucumber roll, California roll, salmon skin roll
ENTRÉES	chicken teriyaki, vegetable or shrimp tempura

what feels right. Some moms-to-be prefer to wait to share the news until they see a heartbeat on the sonogram (around 8 weeks), or at the end of the first trimester (13 weeks), when the babies are less susceptible to miscarriage. Others choose to spill the beans as soon as they test positive for pregnancy, rationalizing that the people they'd tell would be their support network if anything were to go wrong.

"I want to have sex, but my partner is afraid he'll hurt the baby. Crazy, right?"

Before having sex, you should discuss safety with your doc. Although engaging in intercourse while pregnant is usually fine, if you're experiencing any signs of preterm labor (like contractions, or your OB has noticed that your cervix is shortening), you may have to forgo getting busy for the duration of your pregnancy. However, even if you get the green light from your physician that you're good to go, your partner may not be.

Some guys have a tough time with the idea of pregnant sex. First, try assuring him that there is no way a penis (no matter how, um, large) can poke the babies and harm them—or hurt you. The fetuses are safely tucked away in your uterus and surrounded by amniotic fluid. Plus, there's a thick mucus plug that stops germs from getting inside. If he's still not buying it, bring him with you to your next OB appointment and let the doctor speak with him directly.

"Will they grow at the same rate, and if not, how will I know?"

With single babies, an OB can whip out a tape measure and determine a baby's growth just by looking at the size of your uterus. But when there's more than one baby involved, it's more difficult to estimate how much nutrition each one is getting. That's why most moms of multiples get frequent ultrasounds, which are the most accurate way to make sure everyone is doing fine. Most of the time, your tots will be growing at similar, although not identical, rates. Doctors like to see them stay within about 20 percent of each other's weight. Some twins do develop fetal growth restriction, a complication where one baby gains too little weight compared with his sibling with the norm. But the good thing is, your doctor is likely to be on top of your babies' development throughout the pregnancy, so you can address any problems if they should arise.

"What about compared with singleton babies—will my twins grow more slowly?"

Multiples do tend to be born smaller than single babies. But it's not because their growth rate is necessarily slower—in fact, for twins, it's about the same as any other baby's until about weeks 30 to 32, when they do slow down a tad, since they're competing more for nutrients. (Triplets slow earlier—around week 27 or 28.) The real reason multiples are more likely to have low birth

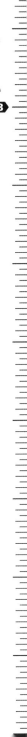

weeks 8–13

weights is that they're more likely to be born preterm (60 percent of twins and 90 percent of triplets are born before week 37).

"It seems like so much can go wrong. How can I know my babies are okay?"
Welcome to parenthood. You're going to worry about your babies for the rest of your life. Literally. So you may as well get used to it now. The truth is, you *can't* know that babies are okay in there. You won't know they're okay with the babysitter, either. Or at college. Yes, there is stuff that can go wrong. But there's a much better chance that everything will be just fine and you're on your way to having healthy little mini-me's. The best thing you can do right now is focus on staying healthy and following your doctor's recommendations. Our advice: Try to stay positive, don't read the scary stuff without a good reason (like if your doctor tells you that you're at risk for something specific), and ban yourself from all of those tragic stories on the Internet. After all, this is a time when you should be celebrating—not stressing.

"What should I do to get my finances and other important things in order before my babies arrive?"
These are important questions, and now is exactly the right time to start thinking about them. (Don't panic, you're not a slacker.) Here's a quick checklist:
HEALTH INSURANCE If you don't have it, get it. Already covered? Read up on your policy so you know exactly what it covers and what it doesn't. This may also be a good time to see what you can deduct from your flexible spending account if you have one—prenatal vitamins and loads of other necessities may be game under your plan.
DISABILITY INSURANCE If you don't have it, you can't get it . . . but your partner can.
LIFE INSURANCE It's not pleasant to think about, but it is important.
SAVINGS PLAN Figure out how much you need to sock away, not just for the birth itself, but really for the next 18-plus years.
MATERNITY LEAVE Bone up on your employer's policy now and start budgeting.
ESTATE PLANNING You may already have a 401(k), but now's a good time to update the beneficiaries if you want. If you don't have a will, talk to a lawyer about drawing up a document. (Yep, another unpleasant topic.) It's also the time to name a guardian for your babies—you know, just in case.

"Is there any way I can tell if they're boys or girls before my big ultrasound?"
There's no way to be 100 percent positive, but there are a number of at-home urine tests you can pick up at the drugstore or mass-market retailers. These tests typically claim 82 to 90 percent accuracy and can be used as early as 10 weeks (6 weeks from your first missed period). That's accurate enough to be fun, but you'll still want to wait until your OB confirms your babies' sexes via an ultrasound at around 18 weeks or an amnio (weeks 15 to 18).

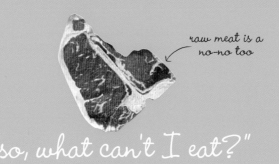

raw meat is a no-no too

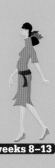

"so, what can't I eat?"

Now that you're eating for three or more, what goes in your mouth is very important. Here's what's off-limits (or partially off-limits) and why.

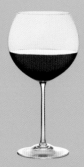

alcohol It goes into babies' bloodstreams and could lead to big problems, from an increased miscarriage risk to issues related to development.

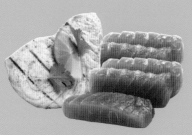

certain fish Stay away from swordfish, king mackerel, tilefish, and shark, which contain high levels of mercury. Any type of raw fish is also a no-no.

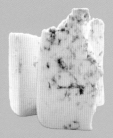

soft, unpasteurized cheese Unpasteurized types, like feta and goat cheese, can contain disease-spreading organisms that put you and your babies at risk.

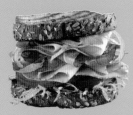

deli meat It could carry listeria, a bacterium that causes serious illness. To play it safe, reheat deli meat to at least 165 °F before eating.

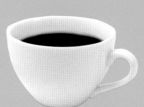

coffee The jury is out on caffeine, but most OBs recommend limiting intake (no more than one or two caffeinated beverages a day) or cutting it out completely.

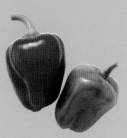

unwashed produce Make sure you clean fruits and veggies to rid them of bacteria.

"what will an early ultrasound be like? how much will I really see?"

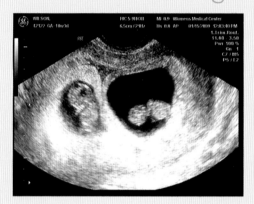

Fraternal boy/girl twins at
10 weeks and 3 days.

This early in the game, your uterus is still way down behind your pelvic bone, so you can't see much with an external ultrasound machine. That means your practitioner needs a more direct route. A transvaginal ultrasound probe (it looks kind of like a dildo and will even wear a condom) is inserted into your vagina (sounds freaky but doesn't hurt). The sound waves it emits form an image of your insides, which appear on the screen for you to see. At this point, your babies will look like small, white jelly beans. You should also be able to tell here if your babies are sharing a gestational sac or are housed in separate sacs, or if they are sharing a placenta. Ask the technician to point out the gestational sac(s) (the membranes that surround your babies), yolk sac(s) (your babies' circulatory systems), and fetal poles (a fancy term for your developing babies, and the first evidence of your embryos). The best part: You may even be able to see the bright, fast flutters of your babies' hearts. Oh, and don't forget to ask for a photo or two to take home!

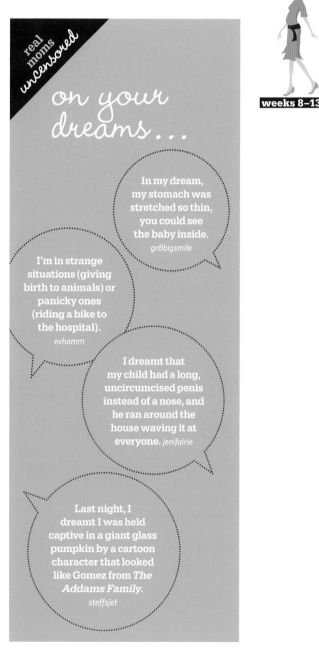

"**I'm sick and sluggish (and I've had to come in late a few times), but I don't want to tell my boss about my pregnancy yet.**"

It does seem cruel that most women feel their worst during the first 12 weeks, when you're trying to keep the news (and your nausea) hush-hush. Until you announce the good news (most people wait until 12 weeks just to be certain everything is okay), there's no milking it for (well-deserved) sympathy. And it's tough to come up with reasons for why you're acting so drained. Here are a few excuses you can try out (not to encourage trickery or anything . . .):

FOR THE SLEEPIES

- I'm fighting a nasty cold and just feel completely wiped out.
- Man, this (yawn) night class I'm taking is really getting to me.
- This kind of weather makes me so sleepy.
- This cold medicine really knocks me out.
- My coffeemaker broke this morning.
- Or put a book on sleep apnea on your desk.

FOR THE LATENESS

- I had to wait for the cable guy/plumber/electrician.
- Argh! I locked myself out of the house again!
- My husband and I are sharing a car while the other one's in the shop. I apologize that it's made me late a few times!
- The traffic's getting really ridiculous—I've got to find a new route to work.
- I can't believe I accidentally set my alarm clock for 7 P.M. instead of A.M.!

real moms uncensored

on your dreams . . .

weeks 8–13

In my dream, my stomach was stretched so thin, you could see the baby inside. *gr8bigsmile*

I'm in strange situations (giving birth to animals) or panicky ones (riding a bike to the hospital). *evhamm*

I dreamt that my child had a long, uncircumcised penis instead of a nose, and he ran around the house waving it at everyone. *jenifairie*

Last night, I dreamt I was held captive in a giant glass pumpkin by a cartoon character that looked like Gomez from *The Addams Family*. *steffsjet*

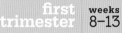
"my boobs are huge...is it maternity bra time, or should I just go up a size?"

Yes, your boobs are changing. When to buy a maternity bra and what to do in the interim? Check out our bra map.

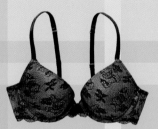

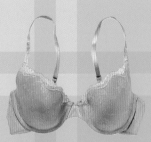

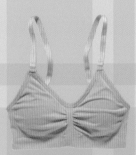

MONTHS 1-3
your regular bra
You can probably get away with your regular bra for the first couple of months. But be realistic and prepare to go up a size soon.

MONTHS 4-6
cheap bigger bra
Hold off on a maternity bra and instead go up in band and cup size. The key: Think cheap. You won't be wearing this bra for long.

MONTHS 7-9
maternity bra
Give in and go for it. A maternity bra gives you major support, especially along your sides, which can get really sore now. Invest in two and rotate them.

the cups just unhook and fold down

POSTBABY
nursing bra
Your goal: support and easy access. Skip the underwire—it puts too much pressure on your breasts and can cause clogged ducts.

POSTBABY
new sexy bra
Your boobs won't be the same—even if your size is back to normal. Now's the time to splurge on at least one sexy new bra.

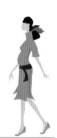

weeks 8–13

"When does my chance for miscarriage drop?"

Most miscarriages occur in the first trimester and are due to chromosomal problems that happen during fertilization. Unfortunately, multiples do carry a greater risk of miscarriage than singletons throughout the entire pregnancy. According to one study where ultrasounds were performed early on in pregnancy, about 9 percent of twin pregnancies result in the loss of both babies, and in 27 percent of twin pregnancies, one of the babies is miscarried. If those numbers seem high, keep this in mind: After week 20, the risks go down significantly, and moms carrying twins have about a 90 percent chance of delivering two beautiful babies.

Most miscarriages involve bleeding and/or cramping. But—and this is important—if you experience bleeding in the first trimester, don't panic; more than half the time it stops and the pregnancy continues to term, so take a deep breath and call your doctor to explain your symptoms. In some cases, there are no warning signs until an ultrasound reveals no heartbeat (this is known as a "missed miscarriage" when the entire pregnancy is lost and as "vanishing twin syndrome" when one of the babies is lost).

"Everyone keeps asking me if twins run in my family or if I had a little 'help.' It's none of their business! But how can I say this politely?"

It's amazing how perfect strangers will have absolutely no qualms about probing into your personal life when you're pregnant. But while it's extremely tempting to fire back an equally intimate question (like "How much weight have you gained since high school?" or "What's your favorite sex position?"), we recommend taking the high road. Smile, explain that you're just excited to be carrying twins, and change the conversation. After all, most people aren't trying to be nasty or intrusive—but at this point in your pregnancy, even the slightest irritant can feel like a major annoyance.

is it normal?

"I. Am. So. Tired. I know this is normal during pregnancy, but is it worse when you're carrying multiples?"

Unfortunately, this is likely a case of bigger not always being better, at least when it comes to the side effects of pregnancy. If you're carrying twins, everything seems to be double—double the hormones, double the stress, double your hunger. And if you're carrying triplets, well, let's just say we completely understand the need for a midday (and morning, and early-evening) nap. It's not just the hormones: Because your body is facing greater demands than even a one-baby pregnancy, you're much more likely to suffer from anemia (iron deficiency), which can make you feel like you've been hit by an 18-wheeler. As tough as it may be in the early stages to stomach the idea of eating anything, let alone eating more of something, try to make sure you're getting enough of those key vitamins and minerals, like iron and calcium. And take your prenatal vitamins—they're like a big old safety net to make sure you're getting at least the minimum amount of the necessary nutrients.

"Is it weird that the doctor only heard one heartbeat, but now, at my ultrasound, he can see twins?"
You may credit your OB with numerous superpowers, but X-ray vision and super-sonic hearing probably aren't among them. Fact is, in the early going it's difficult to hear even one heartbeat until around week 12. So it's not until he starts waving the ultra-sound wand that he's able to get visual confirmation that there's more than one little heart thumping away.

"I suddenly can't sleep! Is this because I'm pregnant?"
Probably. Between the excitement, shock, and hormones, it's no wonder you aren't getting much rest. (Lots of women, whether they're carrying multiples or not, complain of this in the early weeks of pregnancy.) There's no magic solution, but revamping your sleeping environment might help a bit. Start with making the room darker—try blackout liners or heavy drapes. (For a more temporary solution, you could tape up black garbage bags with painter's tape. Ugly, but effective.) Also consider lowering the temp, which helps your bodily functions slow down somewhat, making it easier to rest. The ideal temperature is 68 to 72 degrees Fahrenheit.

Stick a thermometer in your room to double-check it—your thermostat only measures the temp at its own location.

"Why do I have a superhuman sense of smell? When will it go back to normal?"
Crazy, isn't it? You find out you're pregnant, and suddenly you can smell the garbage on the curb of the house three doors down. Like most of your symptoms, hormones are to blame. This is often the worst during the first trimester (as if your nausea needed a boost) and tends to let up (at least a little) as your pregnancy progresses. Explain to your partner why he may want to take up cooking and trash duty for the next month or two, and try to surround yourself with stuff that doesn't reek (try ginger-, lemon-, or mint-scented candles or oils).

"The nausea is killing me! Is there anything that helps?"
Some women get morning sickness (okay, more like all-day sickness) much worse than others. There isn't a magic cure, but there are plenty of things you can try. For starters, don't starve yourself. While eating may sound gross, an empty stomach and low blood sugar can actually trigger nausea. Snack on mini-meals throughout the day, opting for tummy-friendly food, like carbs and yogurt. Steer clear of greasy and spicy foods, which can make nausea worse. Some women swear by saltines. Keep a pack on your nightstand for nighttime sickness, and stash a bag of them in your desk drawer for

midday nausea. Ginger (as in ginger ale and ginger candy) is another excellent option. It has a long history of soothing tummies, and studies have shown that 250 mg taken up to four times daily can help (check with your OB first). Vitamin B$_6$ has been proven to reduce queasiness too—ask your OB if you can take 25 mg tablets up to four times a day. Another secret moms swear by is sour candies. Keep a few on hand during the day. You can even slip on an accupressure band (found at most drugstores) that combats nausea by stimulating acupressure points. People use it for seasickness or car sickness. Finally, keep from getting dehydrated (a nausea trigger) by sipping water and eating hydrating foods, like Popsicles and fruit. If all else fails, check with your doctor about over-the-counter or prescription medications. If you're losing lots of weight or aren't able to keep anything down, seek help ASAP—it could signal a more serious condition.

"Should I be alarmed if I feel cramping?"

Lots of moms have period-like cramps in early pregnancy. As long as the sensations are mild, you (and the babies) are probably just fine. If your cramping is severe, accompanied by bleeding, lasts more than a couple of days, or you just really want to get checked out, go ahead and call your OB.

"I'm not sick and my boobs aren't sore. Should I worry?"

Nope, it simply means you're lucky. Some moms have more obvious symptoms, from morning sickness to constipation, than others. Don't worry—a lack of symptoms doesn't mean anything is wrong with you or your babies. Enjoy feeling normal while it lasts! Oh, and you might want to pretend to feel at least a little bit crappy around other pregnant women just so they don't hate you.

weeks 8–13

"I feel like I pee every five minutes! Why?"

For one thing, the hormone hCG triggers an increase in blood flow to the pelvic area, which makes your body produce more pee. At the same time, your kidneys are kicking into high gear and working more efficiently than ever, so your body gets rid of waste more quickly. And let's not forget your growing uterus, which puts loads of pressure on your bladder as it gets bigger.

The good news is, this pressure lifts once the uterus rises into your abdominal cavity in the second trimester. Until then, be sure to lean forward when you pee to completely empty your bladder. This might cut back on trips to the ladies' room. And even if you're tempted, don't stop downing liquids—your body needs them to stay hydrated.

"Will the heartburn be this bad for the next six months? Will anything help?"

In early pregnancy, progesterone helps the muscles of your uterus relax to stretch for the babies, which also relaxes the valve between your esophagus and stomach. That burning you feel is literally stomach acid bubbling up from your gut. The good news is, heartburn may ease up in the second trimester. But, the bad part: That's also just about the time the babies will begin to squash your digestive organs, causing the same problems. You can't really get that valve to shut again, but you might find some relief by avoiding triggers like chocolate, coffee, tea, citrus, tomato sauces, and spicy and fried foods. It also helps to sleep with your head elevated a bit, and to hold off drinking too much with meals. Just be sure you get plenty of water an hour before and an hour after meals so you don't get dehydrated. The fact is, no matter what you do, you'll probably still feel the burn sometimes. Talk to your doctor about what meds are safe. She'll probably recommend an antacid, like Tums, to start, or something stronger if you're especially miserable.

"What's up with all this saliva?"

Are you also super-queasy? Experts aren't sure why, but women who experience lots of nausea and vomiting also seem to complain about extra saliva. It's probably hormone related. (Plus, nausea can lessen your desire to swallow, making you stockpile your spit.) Luckily, this tends to be only a first-trimester issue—the drool should dry up a bit in coming weeks. Until then, keep hard candy or sugarless gum in your purse (they make it easier to swallow). Some say frequent mouthwash and toothbrushing help, too.

"Why am I getting awful headaches?"

Surging hormones, higher blood circulation, stress, lack of sleep, dehydration, and, hello, caffeine withdrawal can all lead to a pounding head. Luckily, the headaches should go away in your second trimester as your body adjusts to the new hormone levels. In the meantime, get plenty of sleep, exercise, eat healthily, and stay hydrated. If the pain does hit, apply a warm compress to your face or a cold compress to the back of your neck, rest in a dark room, or take a warm shower. If none of these relieve the pain, talk to your doctor about which pain medications are okay to try.

"Help! I haven't pooped in three days!"

Yikes! Constipation is par for the course, but there are some things you can do to help move things along. Fill up on fiber (whole grains, fruits, and veggies) and drink lots (as in eight or more glasses a day) of liquids, especially water. Though you may not feel so motivated right now, exercise can help too. Whatever you do, try not to push too hard when you're trying to do your business. (It can lead to a major case of hemorrhoids.) If your system still can't get regular, ask your OB about using Colace or Metamucil. Don't take any meds or home remedies without asking—enemas, laxatives, or other methods could stimulate labor.

"Is it safe to dye my hair?"

No scientific study has proven whether hair color is 100 percent safe during pregnancy, but most doctors now agree that you can cover your roots and grays (with some restrictions; see following). The potential risks involve the chemicals used in dye entering your system, either through your skin or through the air you breathe. To minimize risks, consider these precautions:

- Wait until after your first trimester, when your babies' vital organs are already developed.
- Choose the earliest salon appointment to minimize exposure to chemicals.
- Ask your stylist to avoid letting the dye touch your scalp.
- Go for highlights rather than permanent or semi-permanent color. Highlight solution is covered in foil and doesn't come in contact with the scalp.
- Ask your colorist about natural henna.
- Talk to your stylist about dyes with little or no ammonia or peroxide.
- If you DIY, be sure to wear gloves and work in a well-ventilated room.

"Is it normal not to feel ready?"

In short, yes. In fact, it would be much stranger if you did feel ready. Parenthood is a big deal when you're expecting one baby, but becoming a parent to multiple children at once can be overwhelming, to say the least. Be prepared for personal questions from nosy (but usually well-meaning) friends and family. When you're pregnant with multiples, people will often assume you used fertility treatments, will wonder how you'll afford to care for your new family, or will voice

concerns about your health. Think a bit about how you want to respond to prying inquiries, so you'll be ready. Take a deep breath, relax, and remember that billions of women have been in your shoes. Your life is about to change, but you'll be fine.

weeks 8–13

"What about spotting? When should I worry about it?"

If it happens in the week or two after you conceived, the spotting could be implantation bleeding. This happens when your fertilized egg starts burrowing into your uterus, and can appear as light spotting anytime between 10 and 14 days after you conceive. Because your cervix is über-sensitive right now, you might notice some bleeding after sex. If this happens, wait to have sex again until you've spoken with your OB. Bleeding can also be a sign of infection in your pelvic cavity or urinary tract, or may simply be a result of the increased blood flow to your cervix. Still, call your OB to discuss any bleeding or spotting. It's probably nothing to worry about, but it could also be a sign of ectopic pregnancy, molar pregnancy, or miscarriage.

"I'm having a lot (and I mean a *lot*) of discharge. Is this normal?"

As long as it is clear or whitish and has a mild smell, and you aren't itching or burning, then yes—it's normal. It's called leukorrhea and is made up of secretions from your cervix and vagina. You've probably seen this discharge before, but it's extra-heavy during pregnancy, thanks to ramped-up estrogen production and blood flow to the vagina. You can't get rid of it, but you wouldn't want to—it's your body's natural way of expelling bacteria that could harm both you and your babies. Invest in a box of unscented panty liners and stay away from tight clothes, scented pads, douches, and any other feminine-care products. Also, stock up on cotton panties—they wick moisture away and are best for keeping you clean and dry. Leukorrhea usually tends to get heavier in the days just before labor hits. If you notice this happening weeks before your due date—or if it's pink or brownish at any time during your pregnancy—give your OB a call right away, because this could be a sign of preterm labor. Also get checked by your OB if, in addition to the discharge, you're itching or burning or notice a strange smell. You may have a yeast infection.

"I've lost weight since finding out I was pregnant. That doesn't seem right."

You're growing babies in your body and yet the scale is slipping—weird, huh? Nausea, vomiting, and other symptoms of morning sickness are even more common among women carrying multiples than in those expecting a singleton. (Doctors aren't sure why, but it likely has to do with the overload of hormones coursing through you.) Your babies don't weigh very much yet, and your recent tendency to lose your lunch can suck a few pounds away early in your pregnancy. (If you haven't been sick and you're losing weight, call your OB immediately.) However, it's important to remember that pregnancy is not the time to drop pounds, and you should make sure you're taking in enough calories and nutrients (see page 25 for nutrition guidelines) to feed your babies and stay hydrated. You should see the numbers on the scale rising soon.

Talk to your OB about your weight and try to combat morning sickness by wearing Sea-Bands and nibbling on saltines. Also, snack on foods that appeal to you, even if they don't seem like the healthiest options; the benefits of nutrient-rich foods won't do you any good if you can't keep them down. It's okay to have chips or ice cream (in moderation) if those are the only munchies that don't have you running to the bathroom. Just make sure to drink lots of water and get back on track with healthful eats once your morning sickness passes.

❚ is it safe?

"Should I be concerned about drinking from plastic bottles?"

There has been concern that exposure to Bisphenol A, or BPA, in extremely high doses may cause miscarriage and birth defects. But the effects are noted with exposures that are more than 400 times greater than you'd experience in daily life. If you're worried, ask your doctor what she considers safe.

"how much weight am I supposed to gain?"

Gaining enough weight during pregnancy is extremely important when you're carrying multiples. Sufficient weight gain can help stave off preterm birth and helps your babies develop and boost their birth weight. However, this weight gain should be slow and steady, and your caloric intake should come from healthful and nutrient-rich foods. Eat five or six times day, and pay attention to the vitamins and minerals you consume.

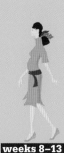

weeks 8–13

TWINS

How much you should gain:

If you're carrying twins and your weight was in the normal range (body mass index of 18.5 to 25) before conception, the American College of Obstetricians and Gynecologists (ACOG) recommends that you gain 35 to 45 pounds during your pregnancy.

When to gain: This means you should be gaining about a pound a week throughout the first half of your pregnancy, and a little more each week throughout the second half.

TRIPLETS

How much you should gain:

If you're carrying triplets, experts advise you should gain between 58 and 75 pounds before delivery.

When to gain: Try to gain the first 35 pounds within weeks 1 through 20.

QUADS

How much you should gain

Moms-to-be of quads should be gaining about 70 to 80 pounds during pregnancy, and because quads tend to arrive around 30 weeks, this weight gain should occur rapidly.

When to gain: Get those numbers on the scale to climb 45 pounds by 20 weeks.

If you were underweight before your pregnancy or you lost weight in the first trimester due to morning sickness, you should try to make up that weight gain as early as possible. If you experience very sudden changes in weight gain or loss, contact your doctor.

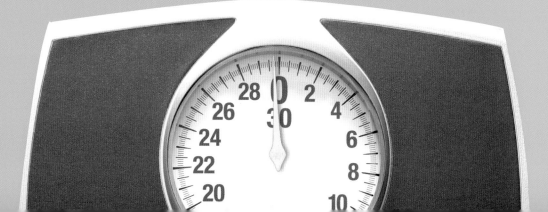

"I heard I shouldn't be in a hot tub while I'm pregnant. Why?"

The problem with a hot tub (or steam room, or sauna) is that it can raise your—and babies'—core body temps too high. There's evidence that temps over 102 degrees could lead to neural tube defects, brain damage, fetal growth restriction, and miscarriage. So nothing super-hot, please.

"Do I have to stop painting my nails?"

Manicures and pedicures have gotten a bad rap because of a certain chemical called dibutyl phthalate, or DBP, that's found in many brands of nail polish. Some experts argue that it can be harmful to your fetus. Others say there's no hard-core evidence that an occasional mani/pedi is unsafe. Your best bet: Choose polish that doesn't have DBP, toluene, or formaldehyde on the ingredient list, and bring it with you to the salon.

"Is it okay to have sex? What about as I get further along?"

If you've got the energy, go right ahead. Intercourse is still considered safe, even when your belly keeps growing. As long as you are not experiencing any signs of preterm labor, like contractions, and your doctor is comfortable with the length of your cervix, sex is safe throughout your pregnancy. (The longer your cervix, the smaller your chance of preterm birth. Your doctor may check your cervix on a transvaginal ultrasound to assess its length.)

However, if you are at risk for preterm labor or miscarriage, or if you notice unusual pain, discharge, or bleeding postsex, your OB may recommend some precautions or restrictions. Sex and orgasms can cause uterine contractions, and depending on your pregnancy, this may be risky.

"What about a vibrator? Is it okay to use one?"

Unless your doctor or health care provider has specifically requested that you refrain from sexual activity, and you aren't experiencing any signs of preterm labor, it's fine to use a vibrator. Make sure that you discuss whether sex is safe for your pregnancy when you visit your OB; because you're carrying multiples, preterm labor is a concern, and orgasms may sometimes cause contractions, so you want to make sure that you're in the clear. However, if your pregnancy is healthy, you and your partner can enjoy a full sexual relationship throughout your pregnancy—with toys!

the day-to-day

"I keep forgetting to take my prenatal vitamins. Is this bad? How can I get into a daily routine?"

It's even more important to get into the swing of taking your vitamins every day once you know that you're pregnant. You need the extra boost of folic acid, calcium, and iron even if you're generally a pretty healthy eater. To jump-start the habit, keep the vitamins

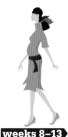

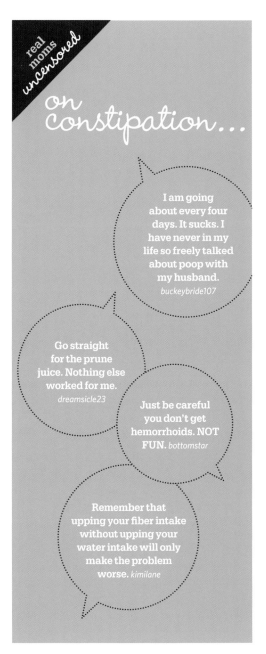

real moms uncensored

on **constipation...**

I am going about every four days. It sucks. I have never in my life so freely talked about poop with my husband. *buckeybride107*

Go straight for the prune juice. Nothing else worked for me. *dreamsicle23*

Just be careful you don't get hemorrhoids. NOT FUN. *bottomstar*

Remember that upping your fiber intake without upping your water intake will only make the problem worse. *kimilane*

next to your toothbrush—you know you'll brush your teeth at least twice a day, so even if you forget the pill in the morning, you'll get another shot at remembering at night. You should also carry some in your purse at all times. That way, when you remember to take them midway through your drive to work, you don't have to head all the way back home or skip them altogether.

"So, I'm eating for three? Do I get to go a little crazy at the vending machine?"
The good news is that when you're carrying twins or more, you do get to add some more to your plate. In fact, a woman of average weight should be taking in about 2,700 calories each day, or enough to gain 35 to 45 pounds (about a pound a week for the first half of your pregnancy, then a little more than a pound a week for the second). But while the occasional milk shake is fine, those babies need their vitamins and minerals, so make those mini-meals well balanced. And don't forget to drink up—it may feel like you're always making a beeline for the bathroom, but it's important to help support the extra blood volume and keep things functioning smoothly.

"Can I exercise just as much as other pregnant women, or do I have to take it easy when carrying multiples?"
While every pregnancy is different, as a general rule, you're going to want to significantly decrease the amount of cardio activity you do when pregnant with multiples. That

"what staples should I have in my closet to get me through my pregnancy?"

☑ *you have*   ☐ *you need*

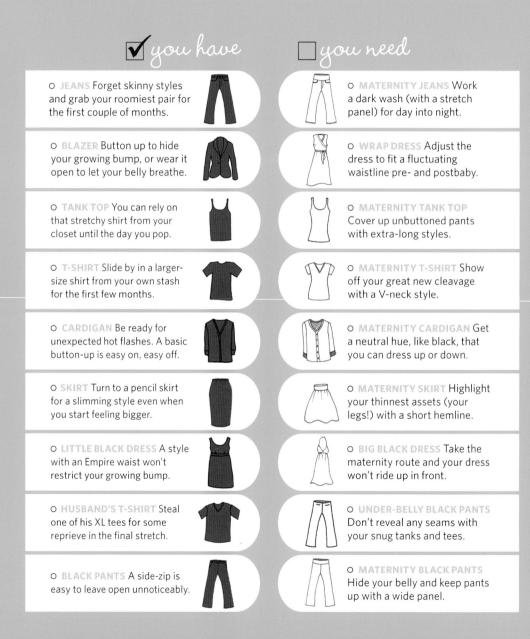

○ **JEANS** Forget skinny styles and grab your roomiest pair for the first couple of months.

○ **MATERNITY JEANS** Work a dark wash (with a stretch panel) for day into night.

○ **BLAZER** Button up to hide your growing bump, or wear it open to let your belly breathe.

○ **WRAP DRESS** Adjust the dress to fit a fluctuating waistline pre- and postbaby.

○ **TANK TOP** You can rely on that stretchy shirt from your closet until the day you pop.

○ **MATERNITY TANK TOP** Cover up unbuttoned pants with extra-long styles.

○ **T-SHIRT** Slide by in a larger-size shirt from your own stash for the first few months.

○ **MATERNITY T-SHIRT** Show off your great new cleavage with a V-neck style.

○ **CARDIGAN** Be ready for unexpected hot flashes. A basic button-up is easy on, easy off.

○ **MATERNITY CARDIGAN** Get a neutral hue, like black, that you can dress up or down.

○ **SKIRT** Turn to a pencil skirt for a slimming style even when you start feeling bigger.

○ **MATERNITY SKIRT** Highlight your thinnest assets (your legs!) with a short hemline.

○ **LITTLE BLACK DRESS** A style with an Empire waist won't restrict your growing bump.

○ **BIG BLACK DRESS** Take the maternity route and your dress won't ride up in front.

○ **HUSBAND'S T-SHIRT** Steal one of his XL tees for some reprieve in the final stretch.

○ **UNDER-BELLY BLACK PANTS** Don't reveal any seams with your snug tanks and tees.

○ **BLACK PANTS** A side-zip is easy to leave open unnoticeably.

○ **MATERNITY BLACK PANTS** Hide your belly and keep pants up with a wide panel.

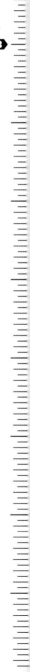

being said, your doctor may very well approve other types of exercise, such as swimming, yoga, and arm exercises. If your regular routine includes walking or the stationary bike, this may also be something you can continue doing during the first part of your pregnancy. Just be sure to check with your doctor first, and avoid exercises that require you to lie flat on your back or jump around too much.

"Is pregnancy brain real?"

Fortunately (or unfortunately, depending on how you look at it), there's no scientific research that proves you get flaky while pregnant. But there are still tons of mamas-to-be who say they feel more forgetful and spaced out. So what's to blame? Hormonal changes, lack of sleep, and/or not being able to stop thinking (and stressing!) about your new babies. Save your sanity by writing down everything, as well as making lists. Regular snacks and getting lots of rest will help you feel a lot more like your old self too. And be sure to take your prenatal vitamins—they contain a number of ingredients that help boost mental sharpness.

"Why am I having *crazy* dreams?"

Dreams reflect your mental state, and let's face it—you're kind of a basket case right now. Hormonal changes—specifically, progesterone and estrogen surges—also contribute to wacky dreams. And don't

forget your constant nighttime awakenings. Dreams come during deep REM sleep, and when you wake during this stage, it's much easier to remember a dream. So why are you dreaming about rainforests and oceans . . . and talking animals . . . and sex (not just with your spouse) . . . and tall buildings? These common themes represent emotions and anxieties about your changing body, the people growing inside you, and your evolving relationship with your mate. Think of it as your subconscious way of working through stress and those heavy emotions.

"When will I start showing?"

This is different for everyone. Your fetuses are pretty tiny in the first few months, so other people won't be able to see much—if any—change in your belly. If this is your first pregnancy, it could be a long while before strangers are asking when you're due. If it's not your first pregnancy, you'll start to show much faster. Also, moms-to-be of multiples are advised to gain more weight and even more quickly than those of singletons, so you may notice changes in your body before your belly actually "pops." By about 12 weeks, when the top of the uterus has grown up and out of the pelvic cavity, you'll probably be able to see and feel it just above the public bone. (But remember, many moms see it even earlier.) This significant change usually signals the beginning of your visible baby bump . . . meaning, time to start browsing the maternity racks!

weeks 8–13

"My clothes are getting tight, but I'm not ready for maternity clothes yet. Any ideas for this in-between stage?"
Hoping to squeeze into your favorite jeans for another week or two or three? The "rubber band trick" is an old favorite of ours: For extra room around the waist, take a regular rubber band or hair elastic, loop it around your pant button, and then thread it through the button hole and loop back around the button. A big safety pin works too. Pull over a long sweater or blouse and no one will be the wiser. Or, grab a belly band. You can find some version at most maternity stores. It's essentially a tube of fabric that stretches over your belly to hold up unbuttoned bottoms or maternity jeans that are too big, support your belly as it grows, and smooth over your "outie" when it inevitably pops. As for tops, dig through your closet for pieces that give you some space. Empire waists and flowing silhouettes will conform to your expanding figure. Raid your guy's closet too, and don't be shy to ask for short-term loans from a one-size-bigger friend. (Pay it forward by offering up your own goods when a pal is pregnant.)

"I'm tempted to buy a Doppler and listen to the baby at home."
You can buy a fetal heart monitor—aka a Doppler machine—from a ton of retailers. (Google "fetal Doppler" and you'll be flooded with results.) Most of these are pretty much the same as what your OB uses, and yep, you can use them to listen for the little ones. They seem to be safe for babies too—just remember you might not find the peace of mind you're after. Sometimes, it can be tough to find fetal heartbeats (and even tougher to find two or more), stressing out many a mama to no end. Our doctor friends have had a ton of calls from women freaked out about changes in the heart rate, too. Keep in mind anything between 110 and 160 BPM is cool.

"I know being super-emotional is part of pregnancy, but how do I deal?"
Blame this one on the hormones! During the first few months after conception, levels of hormones, like estrogen and progesterone, change dramatically, which in turn has a significant effect on brain chemistry (that explains why you're suddenly bursting into tears during dog food commercials). For most women, moodiness is most noticeable in the first few months of pregnancy, then again in the last weeks leading up to delivery and often for a while after their babies are born. If yours seem extreme or are affecting your way of life, bring it up with your doctor. She'll be able to guide you to further forms of care that are safe and effective. But rest assured that what you're feeling is totally normal. Sometimes you just have to stop and remind yourself that it's the hormones talking (or crying or screaming) and not "the real you"!

"I deserve some pampering before my babies arrive, right? Any creative ideas?"
Prenatal pampering is definitely one of the biggest trends around—and rightfully so!

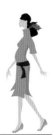

weeks 8–13

Here are some of our favorite ways to treat yourself (and your partner) before diaper changing and 2 A.M. feedings take over:

HIRE A BABY PLANNER They'll help you design a nursery, set up your baby registry, and even send out birth announcements when the time comes. Come on, you had a wedding planner. . . don't your babies deserve the same treatment?

TAKE A BABYMOON With new babies on the way, it's tough to predict the next time you and your husband will be able to get some alone time, let alone an actual getaway. That's why now is such a perfect opportunity to sneak off for a romantic just-for-two vacation. Hotels and resorts offer tons of fun packages exclusively for moms-to-be and their partners. You won't be sorry—guaranteed!

HIRE A PHOTOGRAPHER FOR MATERNITY PHOTOS At first, it may sound like the world's worst idea—pay to document your expanding belly and create a lifelong keepsake?! But trust us: Tasteful maternity photos are the perfect way to capture the innate beauty of your pregnant body and your personality.

GET A FOOD DELIVERY SERVICE It's tough enough to maintain a healthful diet when life is normal. Add the nutritional demands of pregnancy plus your never-ending to-do list, and you've got a perfectly legitimate reason to splurge. Some delivery services even have special menu plans designed specifically for pregnant women, so do your research first. And ask for a taste test before you commit long-term.

"Someone told me I should be lying on my left side more now that I'm pregnant with multiples."
We can't always control the position we sleep in, but it's a great idea to get in the habit of sleeping on your left side during pregnancy if at all possible. This can help improve the flow of blood and nutrients to your body and can even help reduce swelling in your ankles, feet, and hands. If you need to switch positions, the second-best option is sleeping on your right side. Avoid sleeping on your back as much as possible. For one, it's probably going to be really uncomfortable, but it can also potentially lead to problems like dizziness, sleep apnea, snoring, and even a change in blood pressure.

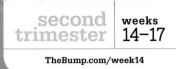

chapter
one trimester down

two

hello, second trimester! Time to pull your head out of the sand (or the toilet) and enjoy the real perks of pregnancy, like chivalry from complete strangers and a cute round tummy popping from under your shirt. Any day now, you should be gaining energy, sanity—and a whole new wardrobe! Your chance for miscarriage has dropped super-low by now, too, so go ahead and spread the big news if you've been holding out. (You'd better hurry before your swelling belly tips them off.)

your to-do list

- Get an amnio

- Boost your calories (again!)

- Look into maternity leave (you may get more because you're having multiples)

▶ **Download our maternity leave checklist at** TheBump.com/matleave

what you're in for…

" my belly feels stretched!

my bump is noticeable.

I finally have energy again.

MASSIVE KICKING

Wow! I think I felt a kick.

the morning sickness is gone.

I NEED NEW CLOTHES.

WHOA, I'M GAINING A LOT OF WEIGHT NOW.

on your mind...

▌at the ob's office

"Is there anything I can do to prevent intrauterine growth restriction?"

Intrauterine growth restriction (IUGR) is a serious condition that happens when one of the babies' weight is below the 10th percentile for its gestational age. While many factors can lead to IUGR, proper nutrition is key to preventing it. The best thing you can do as a mom-to-be is avoid those risk factors that are within your control. They're the obvious things: staying away from alcohol and drugs, quitting smoking, closely monitoring yourself if you have high blood pressure, and making sure you're eating right.

You may hear this referred to as a triple screen or a quad screen, depending on how many of your hormones your OB measures. If administering a triple screen, your doc will monitor your levels of estriol, human chorionic gonadotropin (hCG), and alpha-fetaprotein (AFP). A quad screen includes these, as well as your level of the hormone inhibin-A.

Talk with your OB about which screening is right for you. And remember: As with all other screenings, you won't get any definites. Abnormal results are possible even if your babies are fine, or you may get normal results even if one or more of your children is afflicted. These screenings will simply give you a sense of your risk; these are not simple

weeks 14–17 ▶

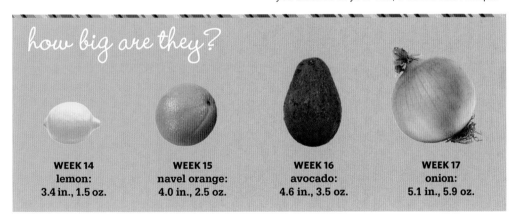

how big are they?

WEEK 14	**WEEK 15**	**WEEK 16**	**WEEK 17**
lemon:	navel orange:	avocado:	onion:
3.4 in., 1.5 oz.	4.0 in., 2.5 oz.	4.6 in., 3.5 oz.	5.1 in., 5.9 oz.

"What is a multiple marker screening, and how do I know if I need one?"

It's a simple blood test that monitors your hormones in order to check for an increased risk of certain conditions like Down syndrome, trisomy 18, and open neural tube defects (spine or brain disorders, like spina bifida).

"yes" or "no" tests. If results suggest a risk, you'll be offered additional testing, like CVS or an amniocentesis, which may diagnose a condition.

The multiple marker screening is accurate only from week 15 through week 20 of your pregnancy, so ask your OB about it at this month's appointment so she can schedule it within the next couple of weeks.

"What happens during an amniocentesis?"

An amniocentesis (often called "amnio") is a test that involves the insertion of a long, thin, hollow needle into your belly to extract about an ounce of liquid from each amniotic sac (the bags of fluid that surround your babies). First, the OB will use ultrasound imaging to find some nice pockets of fluid that her needle can suck up. Once she sticks you, the needle will stay in from 30 seconds to a few minutes (if your babies are not sharing an amniotic sac, you'll have to be stuck again). Most moms say it doesn't hurt too badly. Your doc then sends the fluid on to a lab, where your babies' cells are studied for chromosomal abnormalities, genetic disorders (if you're at risk), and neural tube defects (brain and spine disorders, like spina bifida). If you're interested, this test can also reveal your babies' genders. Amnio results typically take up to two weeks.

Amniocentesis does carry a slight risk of miscarriage (less than 1 percent), so it's not a routine procedure. Your OB is more likely to suggest this if your babies are at increased risk of chromosomal or genetic defects, if earlier screenings suggested potential problems, or if you're over the age of thirty-five. Amnios are generally performed between weeks 16 and 20, but if you're showing signs of preterm labor in your third trimester, your OB may suggest an amnio to determine whether your babies' lungs have matured well enough to function properly outside the womb.

If you're gearing up for an amnio, reduce the risk by checking out your provider's level of experience. If you're referred to a specialist or a testing center, ask about the procedure-related miscarriage rate and how many tests they perform yearly (look for a provider who performs 50 or more). Do the same for the ultrasound technician—experience reduces the risk of injury and increases the chances of getting a good sample in the first attempt.

If you experience severe cramping, begin leaking fluid, or develop a fever after your amnio, call your OB immediately. These may be signs of infection or miscarriage.

"What is a cordocentesis?"

Cordocentesis (aka percutaneous umbilical blood sampling) is a specialized form of testing that can be used to determine if your babies carry certain genetic or blood defects. Cordocentesis tests samples of the babies' blood, pulled from their umbilical cords. It's only when a woman and her doctor agree that the need for information outweighs the risks of the procedure, which include miscarriage, blood loss, infection, and premature rupture of membranes. Usually, that is when chorionic villus sampling (CVS) or amniocentesis test results are inconclusive.

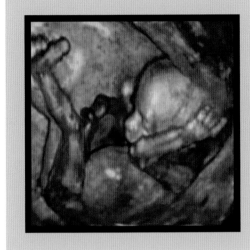

what babies are up to

- thumb sucking
- mastering the art of toe wiggling
- "breathing" amniotic fluid
- liver, kidneys, and spleen continue to develop
- lanugo (thin, downy hair) grows
- joints officially work on all four limbs
- hearing begins to develop
- eyebrows, eyelashes, hair, and taste buds form
- skeleton begins to harden
- finger (and toe!) prints form

weeks 14–17 ▶

▌in your head

"I'm nervous that one of the babies will kick the other in utero and hurt him or her. Does this ever happen?"
Just like singleton babies, twins can sometimes get super-active in the womb. But not to worry; there's no real threat from it. Babies can kick or even hit each other (yes, really) in utero, but the amniotic fluid acts as a cushion to protect them from actually getting hurt by any of it.

"My morning sickness is gone, I'm not so tired, and I don't feel very pregnant. How do I know this is REAL?"
Funny, isn't it? At first you wish for all the nasty symptoms to let up, and then it feels weird when they do. Luckily, feeling good doesn't make you any less pregnant. Stop worrying and try to enjoy your newfound ability to keep your eyes open (and your food down). It's normal to feel a bit strange right now, especially if you aren't showing much or feeling the babies yet. Use all that energy to start planning the nursery, or to organize your maternity leave—or your closet. Get as much as possible done and out of the way while you're feeling good.

"Will I get stretch marks? Is there any way to prevent them?"
Stretch marks pop up on the bellies, bottoms, boobs, or backs of over half of pregnant women. You probably won't see them until your skin starts expanding super-quick in month 6 or 7, and you're more likely to get them if you are carrying multiples. Genetics factor in too.

There's no hard evidence that lotions,

creams, or oils will actually prevent the marks, but moisturizing does seem to help protect skin's elasticity, so it's worth a shot. (These formulas also help tame the itching that can come with stretching skin, so it's a win-win.) Start massaging it in regularly to get your skin ready for the months ahead. Apply after a bath or shower while your skin is still damp to lock in the moisture.

"Will I 'pop' sooner because I'm having twins?"

With twice the baby and twice all the accompanying fluids and placenta growth, there's simply more there to carry. While many moms-to-be first start to show at about 22 to 28 weeks, those with multiples will probably announce their pregnancy to the world by as early as 20 weeks.

❧ is it normal?

"My hair's going nuts. What can I do?"

During pregnancy hormones hit every head in a different way; dry hair may turn oily and curls may straighten. Oh, and that's just the beginning—hair might start sprouting on other parts of your body too!

You know you can't change your hormones (you would have done this weeks ago if it were an option), but you can be extra-nice to your hair and hope it reciprocates. Start with nutrition: Yogurt, fresh fruits and veggies, seeds, and whole grains are especially good for hair. Keep track of the nutrients you're taking in—dry, brittle hair that falls out easily or lightens in color might be a sign of iron, iodine, or protein deficiencies. You can also help undernourished hair by giving yourself a daily five-minute scalp massage to stimulate circulation. Or try an at-home oil treatment (great for fighting frizz). Massage half a cup of warm vegetable or olive oil into your scalp and hair, and let it soak under a shower cap for half an hour or so before washing it out.

> My hair has become so greasy and oily and I have an awful, awful dry scalp. I seriously look like I'm going through puberty again.
> *ernlei608*

"Why are my teeth and gums so incredibly sensitive?"

It's the hormones again, and it's normal—especially in the second trimester. But talk to your OB or dentist if your gums turn bright red, feel really sore, and bleed very easily. These are symptoms of pregnancy gingivitis, which could turn into an even more serious condition called periodontitis if left untreated. (Periodontitis has been linked to premature and low-birth-weight babies.)

To keep your mouth in check, brush and floss at least twice a day (including gums), avoid sweets (especially chewy ones), and up your calcium and vitamin C intake. It may also help to switch to a softer toothbrush.

Go ahead and pay a visit to your dentist early in your pregnancy—just make sure to mention your condition and avoid X-ray exposure. And don't worry . . . your gums should return to normal soon after delivery.

"I feel unattractive since gaining my pregnancy weight and I'm self-conscious about having sex with my husband. Am I crazy?"
This is totally normal. It's easy for women in general (even those who aren't pregnant) to get wrapped up in little insecurities. Multiply that by 10 for you—your body is changing so much right now. It's a lot to get used to. But relax. The truth is, your guy thinks of you in a completely different way than you see yourself in the mirror. He doesn't notice every extra pound. When he looks at you he sees the whole package of the woman he loves. He probably tells you this, but he does want to be with you. So take a deep breath, remember he loves you, and keep reminding yourself what a fabulous mom-to-be you are. If none of this helps, do things that will make you feel better about putting on the extra pounds (as long as your OB says it's okay), like walking or taking the stairs instead of the elevator when you can.

"My belly cramped and got super-hard after I had an orgasm. Should I worry?"
Sexual activity is usually safe while pregnant; just make sure you discuss it with and get cleared by your physician first. It's normal for your uterus to contract when you orgasm; it's always done that. Now it's just a good deal bigger, so you notice it.

Pay close attention to your body; if the cramping is severe, lasts for more than a few minutes, intensifies, or becomes a series of contractions, or if you're bleeding (bright-red blood, not just spotting), call your OB right away. It could signal miscarriage. If you're not experiencing any of these symptoms, just chalk this up to another weird thing that happens during pregnancy.

❚ is it safe?

"I have a long-awaited cross-country trip planned. Is it okay to travel for so long?"
Probably, but you need to discuss it with your doctor. Air travel has been declared safe for most pregnant women before week 32, but remember, all multiple pregnancies are considered high risk. If your pregnancy has gone smoothly and your doc says it's okay, go right ahead. After all, once the babies come, you probably won't be doing a lot of traveling, so enjoy. During the flight, make sure to get up and walk around to avoid deep vein thrombosis (DVT), in which a blood clot forms deep in the vein. Pregnancy increases the risk of DVT, due to your body's natural tendency to prevent excessive bleeding during childbirth. You should also drink plenty of water to combat dehydration, which can trigger contractions.

"What should I do if I get a cold? Is there any chance it can hurt the babies?"
It would be nice if pregnant women were magically shielded from sickness, but it just doesn't work that way. It's totally normal to

weeks 14–17

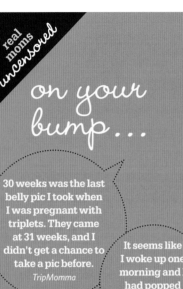

real moms uncensored

on your bump...

> 30 weeks was the last belly pic I took when I was pregnant with triplets. They came at 31 weeks, and I didn't get a chance to take a pic before.
> *TripMomma*

> It seems like I woke up one morning and I had popped overnight. Hello, bump!
> *MrsHT*

> The night before my c-section, I measured 48 inches around. I started off as a size 0!
> *PianoPlayingSarah*

> I never thought I would fit back into my pre-preg clothes, but five weeks after delivering my twins, I'm wearing my jeans again. And now I weigh 12 lbs. less than before I was pregnant.
> *MetalMonkey*

catch a cold or two, and it's not likely to have any effect on your babies. But you do need to keep watch over your symptoms. Some things you normally wouldn't think twice about, like a headache, can actually be a sign of complications. Let your OB know when you're not feeling well. And definitely give her a call before taking any medication—even over-the-counter ones and herbal remedies. Some medicines get the green light during pregnancy, but others can harm your babies. And there are some that are fine on their own but can be dangerous if you combine them. Many OBs will give out a list of meds that they consider safe—keep this stuck to your fridge or in another easy-to-remember place. In general, to help yourself get (and stay!) healthy, you know the drill: Take your vitamins, eat healthy, drink lots of water, and get plenty of rest.

"Is it safe to eat food that's been sitting out on a buffet? How about leftovers?"
The basic rule is that if it's usually served hot, eat it hot. And if it's usually served cold, eat it cold. You're especially vulnerable to bacteria when you're pregnant, so stay away from hot or cold food that's been sitting out at room temperature for two hours or more. If you're at a party and want to go for seconds, reach for safe items like veggies, fruits, and bread. Dying for more mini-meatballs after the two-hour rule? It's okay to pop them in the microwave for a couple of minutes to zap any bacteria that are hanging around. Same goes for other foods that are normally served

hot—a quick zap should keep you safe. As for leftovers, be sure to store them in the fridge and reheat thoroughly.

"I have a very high-pressure job. Can stress have a negative impact on my babies? If so, what can I do?"
The simple, honest answer is that stress is not good for your babies. Studies show that stress during pregnancy can lead to preterm labor and low birth weight. There's even evidence that babies who experience stress in utero are more likely to develop chronic health problems later on.

That said, stress is an inevitable part of all our lives, and only one factor among many in maintaining a healthy pregnancy. The last thing we want is for women to start stressing about the stress in their lives. With work stress, think about ways to take on a lighter load. Now is the time to start wrapping up projects, not take on new ones. After all, maternity leave is right around the corner. So start delegating and crossing things off your list. If a job-share arrangement is an option at your office, consider that as well.

If reducing your workload isn't feasible, there are plenty of tools out there to help manage the stress, including journaling, meditation, prenatal yoga, counseling, and stress-reduction classes. Even getting lost in a book or curling up with a season of your favorite TV show can help ease postwork anxiety. And don't forget to set aside some time for regular, low-impact exercise (our favorite stress-buster) and eat frequent,

small, healthy meals and snacks throughout the day. The healthier your body, the better it will be able to handle the inevitable stress inducers thrown at it.

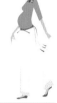

weeks 14–17

the day-to-day

"I am so sick of water. How else can I get my liquids in?"
Water really is the best way to stay hydrated, but other things count too. Even fruits and veggies add to the "8 cups a day" tally. (Five servings of produce = 2 servings of fluid.) And don't forget Popsicles! You may feel like you're going to float away, but don't stop drinking. Instead, think about all the great things downing a glass of H_2O can do: form amniotic fluid, produce extra blood, build new tissue, carry nutrients, help indigestion, and flush out your wastes and toxins (babies', too). Drinking lots of liquids during pregnancy can also ease constipation (and hemorrhoids), soften your skin, reduce edema, and decrease risk of urinary tract infections and preterm labor. Now don't you want to drink up?

"Do I really have to drink five glasses of milk a day? I don't care for the stuff."
There is a loophole: This recommendation is based on your need for calcium, which is (at least) 1,500 mg per day and is nonnegotiable (if you're carrying triplets or more, talk to your doctor—you may need to up this daily dose), but you don't have to get it from milk. The good news is, you can get calcium

from lots of foods; great sources of it are cheese, yogurt, tofu, fortified OJ, tortillas, boiled turnip greens, spinach, fortified bread, canned sardines, and canned salmon. As long as you're getting five servings of calcium a day, it can come from whatever foods you crave. Why so much? Well, your babies' bones have to come from somewhere! In fact, if you skimp on calcium in your diet, your babies will start leaching it from your bones. Not good. Your prenatal vitamin should have about 150 to 200 mg of calcium, and it's a pretty good idea to pick up an extra supplement if your diet needs a boost. Grab one that lists citrate carbonate as the main ingredient—it's the easiest for your body to absorb. And check that the label says "lead free"; some so-called "natural" supplements actually contain lead, which is bad for both you and your babies. Also, remember that caffeine inhibits the absorption of calcium, so this is another good reason to cut down.

"I'm a vegetarian. Can I keep up my diet and still provide my babies with all they need?"

Of course. The main thing to watch out for is your protein intake. But many foods besides meat are rich in protein: eggs, tofu, soy burgers, legumes (beans, chickpeas, lentils, peas), whole grains (eat with legumes for a complete protein), nuts and seeds, milk, soy milk, cheese, fruits and vegetables, and peanut butter (now you've got a good excuse to eat a spoonful straight from the jar!).

Pay special attention to other nutrients usually found in meat too, like vitamin B_{12}, zinc, iron, omega-3 fatty acids, vitamin D, and calcium. And, of course, don't forget your prenatal vitamin!

"I need some ideas to help hide my pregnancy just a little longer."

Hiding the big news can get more difficult as your belly begins to grow, but here are a few fashion tips that might help:

- Wear black—it's the color of disguise. (You may want to keep this up postpartum, too!)
- Choose boxy layers. A suit jacket over a black top offers ideal bump coverage when you're at the office.
- Drape a scarf around your neck and knot it loosely in front to camouflage a growing bust. The V shape it creates will draw the attention up toward your face.
- Keep eyes focused up top with red lipstick, big earrings, or a chunky necklace.

"Do I get more maternity leave since I'm having multiples?"

It certainly doesn't hurt to ask. In many cases, your employer may be willing to give you a little extra time for you to adjust to your growing family, and in some states employers are required to provide extra unpaid leave for women with multiples. At a minimum, though, the Family and Medical Leave Act (FMLA) entitles eligible employees to up to 12 weeks of unpaid leave in a 12-month period when a baby (or two, or three, or more) is born.

"what are some healthy ways I can eat to get in my extra calories?"

To eat 2,700 calories a day is a lot, and it's tempting to fit in extra ones by having some Doritos—but that won't do your babies much good. Try these (roughly) 300-calorie ideas the next time you're reaching for a mini-meal. Since you need to eat 680 extra calories a day in your second trimester, you can have two of these snacks.

weeks 14–17

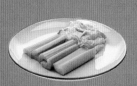

hummus scooped with your favorite assorted raw veggies, like carrots or celery

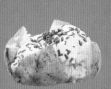

8-ounce smoothie made with your favorite mixed berries, and soy or skim milk

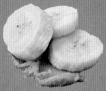

small baked potato topped with plain yogurt (instead of sour cream) and chives

a banana and 1 tbsp peanut butter make it even healthier with all-natural PB

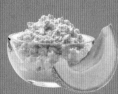

½ cup low-fat cottage cheese with 1 cup of fresh fruit dropped on top

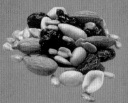

dried fruit and nuts just a small handful has plenty of healthy fats and proteins

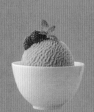

1 cup of sorbet or vanilla ice cream topped with fresh fruit

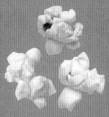

popcorn 6 cups of the air-popped kind with ¼ cup parmesan cheese

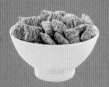

1 cup whole-grain cereal mixed with soy or skim milk for breakfast anytime

¼ cup salsa paired with two handfuls of your favorite baked tortilla chips

avocado cut one-fourth of one and spread it out onto eight whole-grain crackers

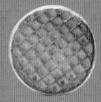

whole-grain waffle right out of the toaster and with peanut or almond butter on top

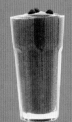

chapter

bump alert

three

welcome to the fun stuff! This month, your bump will start seriously taking shape, bringing on smiles from strangers (hopefully no unwanted belly-pats) and a better fit to your maternity clothes. You may even be forced to go shoe shopping (poor you) as your feet grow about half a size. If you haven't felt your babies kick yet, you will start to do so any day now, and you'll probably get a peek at their tiny profiles during your midpregnancy ultrasound—this also means you may find out your babies' genders this month, making it a good time to narrow down names, register for gifts, start shopping, and get the nursery under way.

your to-do list

- **Have midpregnancy ultrasound**
- **Register for gifts**
- **Think about the nursery setup**
- **Decide on (and agree on!) favorite names**

Search 1,000s of fantastic names at TheBump.com/names

what you're in for...

" My skin is so dry and itchy.

so swollen

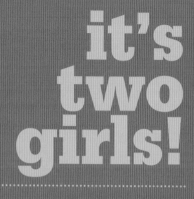

it's two girls!

My bump finally exceeded my boobs.

eating constantly.

feels like I'm carrying two giant cantaloupes

WHY IS MY PULSE RACING?

WTF WAS THAT? CAN THE BABIES KICK EACH OTHER?

my back hurts a lot.

I can see them!

"

on your mind...

▌ at the ob's office

"What will our big ultrasound be like?"
Your midpregnancy ultrasound will happen between weeks 18 and 20 and is usually a "level two" ultrasound (meaning it's pretty detailed). By this time, your OB has already taken a look at your little ones and determined chorionicity, so this time around the technician will be digging a little deeper.

Every office does this differently, but generally it goes something like this: You lie back and the ultrasound technician glops some gel on your belly (if you're lucky, it will have been warmed first) and rubs a wand-like device on your bump. Then your adorable babies' images pop up on a screen!

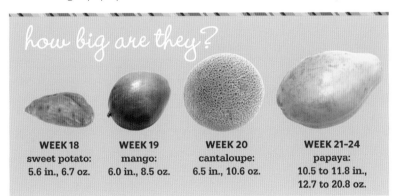

how big are they?

WEEK 18	WEEK 19	WEEK 20	WEEK 21-24
sweet potato:	mango:	cantaloupe:	papaya:
5.6 in., 6.7 oz.	6.0 in., 8.5 oz.	6.5 in., 10.6 oz.	10.5 to 11.8 in., 12.7 to 20.8 oz.

You may be able to watch as the tech searches for the fetal heartbeats, locations, breathing, and movements; placental locations and size; and the amount of amniotic fluid. The technician will also take a bunch of measurements and check for abnormalities. Your cervix will also be checked to ensure it is nice and long, and that you're not at risk for preterm birth. And—if you're interested and the babies are cooperative—the technician can tell you your babies' genders. (Let the shopping begin!)

You'll probably have a follow-up chat with your OB to discuss your babies' status, and you'll walk away with your first pic! Tip: Buddy up with the tech, and she'll likely put more effort into snagging a great shot.

"What's placenta previa?"
Placenta previa is a rare condition where the placenta partially or totally covers the cervix. This can be dangerous when the cervix starts opening in preparation for labor, because it forces the placenta to detach, leading to bleeding. Nearly all cases of placenta previa are identified early these days, either during a routine ultrasound or when a mom-to-be complains of bright-red bleeding in her second or third trimester. If you're diagnosed with placenta previa, tell any doctor you see during pregnancy, even your primary care physician. They'll want to avoid any prodding near your cervix. (If you were wondering, yes, sadly, this means sex is out too.) The good news is that your placenta may move in later months. In fact, in most cases, the placenta slides out of the way well before delivery.

weeks 18–22 ▶

Your OB will probably do a few ultrasounds to track the position of your rogue placenta. If it sticks around the cervix farther into pregnancy, you may have to be put on bed rest or given other lifestyle restrictions to avoid bleeding. One thing to note: If you've got placenta previa that continues late into your pregnancy, your OB will schedule you for a c-section before your cervix has a chance to dilate and cause trouble for either you or your babies.

> At my 3-D ultrasound the tech warned that baby would still look somewhat skeletal. Honestly, I think she looked beautiful. We got a great profile shot and you could already see her features. *BottomStar*

"What's an anterior placenta?"

"Anterior" means "front." If you've been told you have an anterior placenta, it simply means it's located in the front of your uterus, closest to your belly instead of in the back ("posterior"), which is more common. What does this mean for you? Nothing huge, really. Amniocentesis can be a little more challenging with a placenta up front, but in general, an anterior placenta doesn't pose any serious threat to either you or your babies.

"What's up with 3-D ultrasounds?"

All ultrasounds use sound waves and not radiation to take a snapshot of your fetus. A 2-D ultrasound allows you to see a simple cross-section profile, while a 3-D ultrasound looks more like a real photo, with a three-dimensional rendering of your baby's body. The image is achieved by sending sound waves at different angles and by collecting more detailed data to show depth and volume. A 4-D ultrasound takes it a step further and, much like a video, collects images over time—so you will actually get to see your little ones moving around in your belly in real time (making faces, kicking, sucking their thumbs, the works). It's fun—and most moms want to do it at least once to sneak a peek—but don't make a monthly habit out of it.

in your head

"What can I say when people ask me how much weight I've gained?"

Funny how people somehow think this is an appropriate question, right? If you don't feel like sharing the poundage, evade the question. Here are a few phrases that might help.

- "Oh, enough! This baby sure likes chocolate."
- "So far, so good—the doctor says I'm right on track with her expectations."
- "Not as much as I thought I would. I think the yoga classes are helping."
- "Ha. You can really tell the baby's growing, right? It's started kicking now too."

Resist the urge to dig back with, "I see you've gained weight too. How much?" Tempting, we know—but not so nice.

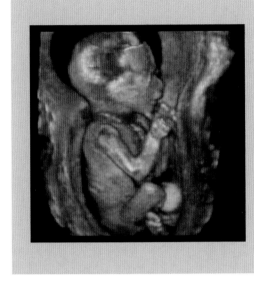

what babies are up to

- yawning and hiccuping
- flipping, twisting, and kicking
- sucking and swallowing
- creating meconium (the stuff that will fill babies' first diapers)
- vernix caseosa (greasy white stuff) covers the skin
- genitals are fully formed
- taste buds work
- eyelids and eyebrows are well developed
- fingernails cover the fingertips

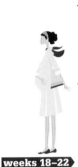

weeks 18–22

"Will my body ever be the same?"

No, not likely. But that's okay. Your body is an amazing thing, designed to be stretched and pulled. The skin on your middle may never be as firm, and you could wind up with stretch-mark souvenirs. But you'll probably also gain some sexy curves. Take good care of yourself now by eating well, and remember that you're supposed to be consuming enough calories per day to nourish your babies. Pregnancy is not a time for dieting; your primary job is to grow healthy babies, so stay within the advised weight-gain ranges. If your doctor says that it's safe for you to exercise, maintain a prenatal regimen throughout pregnancy and keep it up postpartum, and you'll be able to tone up and slim down. Don't expect to drop the "baby weight" overnight, though. Your body is going through 9 months of changes, and it will take another 9 to 12 months to get back into gear.

"I'm swelling. I know this is normal, but when should I worry?"

You're right that it's normal—nearly all pregnant women swell up at least a little, particularly in the feet and ankles. Annoying? Yes. Dangerous? Not usually. However, pay close attention to your body: If your face or hands puff up at all or if your feet and ankles swell severely, call your doctor. Moms expecting multiples are at an increased risk for preeclampsia, and these symptoms may be warning signs. Also alert your physician if one leg is much more swollen than the other, which can sometimes signal a blood clot.

is it normal?

"Why is my skin itchy? And what can I do to make it stop?"

It's normal for your belly and boobs to itch like crazy as your body grows to accommodate babies. All that skin stretching is the culprit— it really dries things out. Your best bet is to dress in soft, comfy clothes and grease up with lotions, creams, or oils. Go for unscented stuff; it's less likely to irritate. Try applying them right after a shower while your skin is still damp to lock in the moisture. Colloidal oatmeal baths are also great for relieving the itchies and soothing skin. (A good thing to remember if you wind up with a rashy baby.) You can make your own if you grind the heck out of oats with a coffee grinder (essentially to powder form) and drop a couple of cups' worth into a warm bath. Or just pick up some oatmeal bath from your local drugstore. And when you bathe or shower, remember to keep the temp lukewarm. Hot water can have a drying effect. (Not to mention, you don't want to overheat.) If your skin starts itching all over (not just your abdomen), let your OB know. This could signal a more serious problem.

"No one told me I'd have varicose veins in my . . . vulva! Is there anything I can do?"

Your veins are working overtime right now thanks to your expanding uterus, increased blood volume, and crazy hormones. And in the spots that are under the majority of the pressure, including your legs, vulva, and rectum (sorry), blood can accumulate. The

real moms uncensored

on names . . .

Whichever twin is born first will be getting the name that comes second alphabetically. That way I can counter any "I'm older!" fights with "Well, your sister's name comes before yours in the alphabet!" *eyelovemascara*

We named the twins after our grandfathers. We decided that the "older" twin would have the same name as the older grandfather. *Aussie's_Mom*

We had difficulty picking two same-sex names to begin with. Even after they were born we hadn't decided on two names we liked. We looked at each baby and assigned names based on the names' meanings and the differences we noticed between the babies in utero. *Caden*

result: swollen, or varicose, veins. So, that's the bad news, but on the bright side, aside from some throbbing here and there, they're pretty harmless and will probably disappear after delivery. To keep them under control (or prevent them in the first place), do things to improve your circulation. Prop your legs up as often as you can, exercise, avoid tight shoes, and try sleeping on your left side so your uterus doesn't press on the vena cava, a major vein on your right side (tuck a small pillow between your legs to take the pressure off your lower back, though).

"Is it possible that I could have developed a third nipple from being pregnant?"
Ummm, the short answer: yes. But it was probably there before and the changes in your breast tissue have simply made it more noticeable. Don't worry, you're not a freak—it's pretty normal, even if it seems weird.

is it safe?
"Are any spa treatments off-limits?"
Sounds like a treat—and one that you clearly deserve! First, research the spa: Call and speak to someone to ensure that the facility and employees have experience treating pregnant women. Be completely up-front with the staff about your pregnancy and how far along you are. Some spas actually offer packages for pregnant women that include specialized massages and intense foot rubs. Avoid heat treatments, like saunas, hot tubs, tanning beds, and body wraps, because

increased body temperature can harm the babies. Also, make sure that none of the treatments require you to be flat on your back, because that position is a no-no this far along in your pregnancy. If you're getting a massage, lie on your side or have the masseuse use a special table with a cutout for your bump.

If your skin is super-sensitive right now, steer clear of facials or look for treatments that use natural and hypoallergenic products. Whatever treatment you choose, make sure your aesthetician is aware of your bump. And, as a rule of thumb, it's always a good idea to check with your OB to make sure she is okay with your blissed-out plans.

weeks 18–22

the day-to-day
"When will I feel the babies kick? And what exactly will it feel like?"
It won't be long! Most first-time moms feel movement at some point between 16 and 22 weeks. If this is your first pregnancy, if you have an anterior placenta (in the front of your uterus), or if you are overweight, it may be a bit later than 22 weeks. Some moms feel what they call "flutters" or "bubbles"; this is a gentle, wave-like sensation, but everyone experiences it differently. You may notice the kicking only if you're sitting or lying quietly. And don't worry too much if your pregnant friends feel kicks sooner than you—those early kicks can be difficult to distinguish from the other weird stuff going on in your belly, like gas, and they can be pretty infrequent.

"My partner hasn't felt the babies kick. How can I help him feel it?"

Like just about everything else, this one's slightly different from woman to woman (and pregnancy to pregnancy). You may have started feeling the babies dance around in there, but it usually takes a little longer for the jabs to be felt from the outside. Most moms say others are able to feel their babies kick sometime between 20 and 30 weeks. Once you start to feel the babies' little knees and elbows jabbing the surface of your belly, you can give your partner a heads-up about times when your babies are particularly active, like just after you drink a glass of cold milk, or when you lie down at night. Cuddle up with his hand resting gently on your tummy, and sooner or later (he'll have to be patient, of course) he just may feel a little thump!

"It's girls (or boys)—or a boy and a girl! How should we go about sharing the news?"

It's always exciting to announce what your babies' genders are! Here are a few fun ideas:

• Buy "I love Grandma [or Grandpa]" onesies in blue or pink, and give them as a gift.
• Walk in wearing a maternity tee that spells it out ("They're girls!" or "They're boys!").
• Invite everyone over to watch a video of the ultrasound and guess the babies' sex. After, have one guest open a gift that reveals the truth.
• Order custom fortune cookies with the big news hidden inside.

• Order a cake with pink or blue frosting inside—the first slice reveals your babies' sex!

"How can I track my belly as it grows?"

Your doctor keeps track of the growth of your uterus by measuring from the top of your pubic bone to the top of the fundus of your uterus. However, it isn't so accurate to try at home. The OB is more experienced in feeling the difference between the top of your uterus and your other insides. Plus, other bump-watching methods are way more fun! Try taking a picture of yourself in profile every day or once a week (stand in the same spot and wear tight clothing). Then, combine the pictures into a flip book or digital slideshow, and you won't believe how much your body is morphing! (This makes a great keepsake of your pregnancy.) Some moms also like to track belly growth by measuring their used-to-be waistlines and then recording weekly measurements in the baby book or a pregnancy journal. You'll rack up a lot of inches in the weeks to come!

"What size clothes should I buy for my newborn baby?"

Aside from your OB's estimation (which can sometimes be way off), there's no way to know what clothing will fit your babies on day one. However, if you're pregnant with multiples, it's pretty likely your babies will be born small; the average birth weight for twins is 5½ pounds, triplets are typically

nursery

change up Convert any dresser into a changing table: Screw in a safety railing around the perimeter and add a plush pad.

crib notes Choose a firm mattress that fits snugly in your crib.

trash talk A small pail with a lid is all you really need for diaper disposal. Just empty daily.

underfoot Spills and messes are inevitable: Choose durable flooring and add rugs.

about 4, and quads generally weigh in the 3-pound range. It may depend on brand, but newborn clothes are generally made for babies up to 8 pounds, so those will likely be too roomy for your little ones. To make matters even more complicated, there is no real standard for "preemie" sizes in clothing, so even clothes that are labeled this way may be too big. You can find small sizes at specialty stores and companies; when you're shopping, just buy a range of sizes and make sure you hang on to your receipts and leave on the tags. Once your babies are born, you can send friends to return any clothes you don't need. Remember, you may want to keep some of those larger clothing items; they will come in handy when your little babies grow big quickly! Don't stress too much about what your babies will wear in those first few days anyway. They don't do much more than sleep and eat, so a few basic onesies or baby T-shirts will do the trick nicely.

"Who's supposed to throw me a baby shower? And when should it be?"

There's no hard rule here: A shower can be hosted by whoever feels like honoring your babies-to-be. Often this is a close friend, a neighbor, a colleague, or, yes, even an aunt, mom, or sister. Sometimes a group of friends and family will pitch in together to host your shower, splitting the costs, cooking, and doing other party prep. Traditionally, it was considered bad form for a family member to host, but that advice has become a little outdated. So if a family member offers to throw you a shindig, it's okay to accept. But don't throw yourself a shower. As for your timing, months 6 through 8 are ideal. Before then, your bump may be MIA (a bigger belly makes for the cutest keepsake pics), and in month 9 you'll be getting uncomfortable. Plus, well, your babies could pop out any minute. We know plenty of moms who tried cutting it close to their due date and wound up with a week-old baby in tow at their showers!

"When should I register?"

If you haven't started a registry already, go ahead and get it going. Your shower hosts will probably want to include your registry information on the invitations. Plus, it can take some time to scope out your ideal gear. (Use our checklist on page 73 to help you determine what you need, and then log on to TheBump.com/registry to start your list.) Just be careful registering for clothes—if your shower isn't happening for a month or two, it's likely the items you choose will already be out of stock when folks start shopping.

"We can't settle on the right name! Where can we find ideas?"

Besides flipping through name books and playing with online naming tools (time for a shameless plug: We have a fun one at TheBump.com!), try simply keeping your eyes and ears open as you go about your day. Read the credits after the movies you watch, check out the captions under

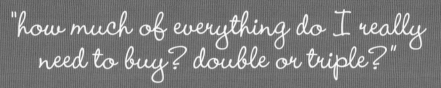

"how much of everything do I really need to buy? double or triple?"

When you consider that buying at least two of everything means you'll be spending twice as much, a budget can get blown pretty quickly. But you don't have to double up on everything.

weeks 18–22

Nonnegotiable doubles:
- Infant car seats. Sorry, need one per customer here, no matter what. Most hospitals won't let you bring your babies home without them.
- Cribs. In many cases you can get away with sharing a single crib for a few weeks, but eventually your little guys are going to want to spread out. For safety—and comfort—give them their own sleeping space when they're starting to move.

Double bonuses:
- Bouncy seats. Those babies aren't going to spend their whole day in the crib, so when it's time to get up, it's nice to have a place to put them. Placing each one in a bouncy seat can give you time to do something fun, like brushing your teeth and doing the dishes.
- Bottles. Even if you plan on breastfeeding, there's a chance you'll have to "top off" with some formula, or you'll have to pump and let someone else do the feeding. Keep those bottles at the ready for when you need them.

One is enough (for now):
- Stroller. Technically, you only need one, but make it a double.
- Twin feeding pillow. Oh-so helpful when it comes to either breast- or bottle-feeding, because you can get double the job done in half the time.
- Play mat. Spending some time on the floor will help your tots develop muscle tone and strength, and you can keep them both on a mat for company.
- Swing. One more place to put 'em down (together if they're small enough, or separately when they get bigger).

photos in the paper, and listen up when you're waiting in line at the store. (Just try not to be too creepy about it.) We know one mom-to-be who searched her company's international e-mail directory for inspiration and another who scoured the shelves at her local bookstore looking out for authors with interesting names. If you're stuck, brainstorming works well too. Sit down with your partner and jot down all the names that come to mind (favorite teacher, great-grandpa, the cute kid in that summer blockbuster . . . anything goes). Don't stress about it—babies don't really need names until you leave the hospital. Plenty of parents make the final call on delivery day. Take your time and find a name that fits your new family to a T.

"When is a good time to start putting together my nursery?"

Most of our pregnant pals say they're aiming for the second trimester. After all, this is the time in pregnancy when you'll feel most up to it, and decorating plans may become more clear if you're peeking at your babies' sex. So get to work! Even if you aren't quite ready to start painting, it's best to go ahead and pick out the major furniture in the next month or so—it can take several weeks to arrive and most likely more than one trip to the store to pick it out. Make sure to measure your nursery before you head out to shop, and bring a tape measure with you to the store so that you know the things you pick out will fit into your babies' room.

"How can I stay comfortable when I have to travel?"

If you're feeling good, your pregnancy is healthy, and you've got your doctor's blessing, the second trimester can be great for traveling, as long as you take a couple of precautions. Circulation is key. Get up and walk around at least once an hour, and wiggle and/or massage your legs every few minutes while sitting. (Same goes for any time you're seated for an extended period of time while pregnant.) Keeping your blood flowing reduces the risk of developing throbbing varicose veins, thrombosis (blood clots), and swollen feet and ankles. Wear your seat belt across your thighs and tucked below your belly. Prop your feet up to help blood flow. If you're flying, request an aisle seat in the front half of the plane. This will give you a smoother ride and make it easier to get up and walk around frequently throughout the flight. Also try using a carry-on item stashed under the seat in front of you or put your feet up on an available seat. Avoid travel-induced dehydration by loading up on noncaffeinated fluids. When traveling by car, push your seat back as far as possible to get more legroom. And, of course, make sure you stop for bathroom and stretching breaks along the way. Request extra pillows wherever you stay. It's not always practical to pack your oh-so-cozy body pillows, so make sure you have enough to sleep comfortably. If you're prone to motion sickness, wear Sea-Bands. Bring nonperishable snacks like nuts, crackers, and granola bars to quell hunger.

checklist

"what should I register for...really??"

Baby stores have huge lists of things to buy. Here's what you really need.

furniture/bedding

- Cribs (your babies may be able to share in the beginning, but they start wriggling around pretty quickly)
- Crib mattresses (1 per baby) and covers
- 2–3 fitted crib sheets (per crib)
- Dresser (depending on how many babies you have, you may be able to fit all of their stuff in 1 large dresser)
- Changing table

gear

- High chairs (1 per baby)
- Swing (buy 1 and see if you need more down the line)
- Bouncer seat or rocker (you may be able to get away with having just 1 here, too)
- Car seats (1 per baby/no skimping here!)
- Car window shade
- Stroller (choose one that can accommodate all of your babies)

- Umbrella stroller (You only really need one stroller, but it's good to also have an umbrella stroller for travel.)
- Baby slings or carriers
- Diaper bag
- Changing mat (just get 1 of these)
- Diaper pail and liner
- Activity mat (get a big one that can accommodate all of your babies)

safety/health

- Baby monitor
- Pacifiers
- Thermometer
- Nasal aspirator
- Baby nail clippers
- First-aid kit
- Infant bathtub
- 2 hooded bath towels per baby
- 4 washcloths per baby
- Baby shampoo and wash
- Brush and comb set
- Diaper rash cream
- Diapers (start with at least 2 cases of newborn size)

layette/clothing

- 4–6 undershirts per baby
- 4–6 receiving blankets per baby
- 4–6 long-sleeved onesies per baby
- 4–6 footed outfits per baby
- 4 sleep sacks per baby
- Caps/mittens

feeding

- Breast pump
- Multiples nursing pillow
- 4–8 bibs per baby
- Burp cloths
- 10–16 bottles per baby (Seem like a lot? Babies go through these very quickly. You'll be happy when you aren't spending your days washing out plastic bottles.)
- Insulated bottle tote
- Bottle brush
- Bottle sterilizer
- Bottle warmers
- Dishwasher caddy

weeks 18–22

chapter

the real kickoff

four

still feeling good? Take it slow and enjoy these last weeks of the second trimester: Your bump's getting big, your babies are kicking up a storm, and you're still mobile enough to get around (pretty) easily. You might be feeling a little more in tune with your babies now that their somersaults are consistent. Go ahead and have a chat with those adorable little aliens growing inside you and play your favorite music—babies' ears are well developed by week 24. Now's also the time to start thinking seriously about your birth plan and figure out what you want (and don't want) to happen when you go into labor.

your to-do list

- Schedule a glucose tolerance test
- Prepare a birth plan
- Take maternity photos

Get the 411 on baby registries at TheBump.com/reg101

what you're in for...

" **THEY'RE KICKING LIKE CRAZY.**

I have an outie now.

holy #!*?— hemorrhoids!

hmm . . . I don't remember that—what's it called again?

I DON'T CARE THAT I'M WEARING SNEAKERS WITH A SKIRT— I'M COMFORTABLE.

I have gas. A lot of it.

I'M SO HUNGRY.

INSANELY. ITCHY. BELLY. "

on your mind...

▌at the ob's office

"I've heard that 24 weeks = viability. What does this really mean?"

Generally, 24 weeks is the earliest that most OBs think your babies have a chance of surviving in the outside world. This means that if you were to go into preterm labor that couldn't be stopped—or if your babies were otherwise in serious trouble and had to be delivered—after you've hit week 24, your babies would have a shot at making it. But your babies would definitely be in for a long stay in intensive care, and would be at high risk for serious problems down the road.

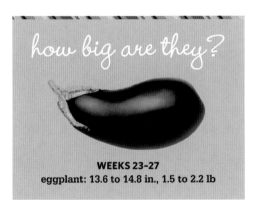

how big are they?

WEEKS 23-27
eggplant: 13.6 to 14.8 in., 1.5 to 2.2 lb

"What's the glucose tolerance test like? What do the results mean?"

The glucose tolerance test (done between weeks 24 and 28) is part of the screening for gestational diabetes. This is especially important for you, since women carrying multiples are at greater risk for it (up to 6 percent of women carrying twins, and up to 39 percent of women carrying triplets).

The test takes one hour and works like this: At your appointment, you'll chug a cup of incredibly sweet, syrupy liquid (it's called Glucola and contains 50 grams glucose). Then you'll wait an hour, after which a sample of your blood will be taken to assess how your body reacts to the glucose. If the results are negative, you're done. If they're positive, you'll need to schedule another screening, called the 100-gram oral glucose tolerance test, for which you'll be tested four times over a three-hour time span. (Bring a book.) Lots of women fail the first test and pass the second with flying colors, but if two out of the four test results show an abnormality, you'll be diagnosed with gestational diabetes and will need to talk with your OB about a health plan for the rest of your pregnancy.

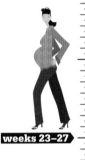

weeks 23-27

"What's preeclampsia?"

Preeclampsia (also known as toxemia or pregnancy-induced hypertension) is a condition where you have a rapid rise in blood pressure and the presence of protein in your urine during pregnancy. It usually develops after week 20 and is especially prevalent among women carrying multiples. In fact, a whopping 1 in 5 multiple pregnancies is diagnosed with preeclampsia—and if you're carrying more babies, your risk is even higher. The cause is still a bit of a mystery, but the consequences are clear: Blood vessels constrict and reduce blood flow, which can affect the liver, kidneys, and brain. The blood flow to your babies may also be interrupted, which—in severe cases—can lead to poor growth, insufficient amniotic fluid, or the placenta (or placentas) peeling away from the uterus. There seems to be a genetic link, so pay special attention to warning signs if your mom had it. Certain conditions you may have suffered before pregnancy can make you more susceptible to preeclampsia, like chronic hypertension, blood-clotting disorder, diabetes, kidney disease, certain autoimmune diseases, and if you're overweight, older than 35, or younger than 20.

Keep a close eye on changes in your body and let your doctor know if your hands, face, or feet swell excessively (for feet, beyond what's normal for pregnancy) or if you gain more than a pound per day. Some other indicators are severe headaches, blurry vision, intense upper abdominal pain, nausea, and vomiting. If you're diagnosed, your doctor will monitor you closely and limit your activities, and may put you on bed rest or induce labor early. Preeclampsia typically goes away once you give birth. There are certain things you can do to lower your risk while pregnant; talk to your doctor about raising your consumption of calcium, which may help combat this condition.

"What are Braxton Hicks contractions? When do you they start?"
Braxton Hicks contractions are relatively painless contractions of your uterus that may begin as early as week 6 (though you won't feel them until around midpregnancy,

and some women don't notice them at all). Some mamas-to-be say it feels like your stomach is squeezing and getting hard, or inflating like a balloon. Sometimes these contractions will go away if you drink a big glass of water (dehydration triggers contractions) or take a warm bath. The important thing for a woman pregnant with multiples is to be able to distinguish between Braxton Hicks and preterm labor. If you have any concerns, call your doctor immediately to discuss your contractions; she may want to check you out to monitor the frequency and intensity of your contractions and to watch for shortening of your cervix, which indicates the onset of labor. Be particularly watchful if you have more than 6 uncomfortable contractions an hour, if the pain is intense, if you have a lower backache, or if there is any change in your vaginal discharge. Don't be shy about contacting your doctor—it's always better to be safe.

in your head
"Can I have a midwife? How about a doula?"
Some moms-to-be choose to have a midwife instead of an OB for prenatal care and to deliver their babies—midwives can deliver babies in hospitals, birthing centers, or even in your home. But here's the biggest difference between OBs and midwives when it comes to multiples preganancies: OBs are surgeons who perform c-sections and midwives are not. Since you're carrying multiples, you're at

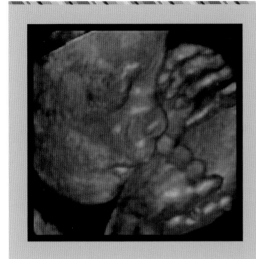

what babies are up to

- little ears develop
- faces are fully formed—minus the baby fat
- skin is becoming more opaque
- babies are learning to distinguish right-side up from upside down
- eyes are forming—soon they'll be trying out their blinking skills

weeks 23–27

increased risk for preterm birth, preeclampsia, and needing a c-section, so it's probably a better idea to go with a doctor who will deliver your babies in a hospital and can respond quickly if you need surgery. Be sure to interview any health care practitioners you're considering thoroughly and ask lots of questions about your particular needs and their experience in delivering multiples. As for a doula, she's essentially a labor coach, and you can hire one no matter what—she'll help you get through labor and delivery but isn't a substitute for an OB or midwife.

"Any tips for do-it-yourself maternity picture poses?"
Hey, you're the artist. Think about how you can use the photos to communicate how you've been feeling. Had a wacky dream? Use it as inspiration. Craving certain foods?

Balance them on your belly. Just felt like your belly finally "popped"? Go in for a close-up. You can also use the camera to try and capture other stuff that's going on in your life during your pregnancy—try incorporating your pets, other children, and, of course, your partner.

"I think I'd like to change my work schedule after my babies. Should I talk to my boss about it now? How?"
If you're hoping to switch things up once your maternity leave is over, it is probably best to lay your ideas on the table now. First, make sure you're clear on what your company's policies state (like whether part of your leave would be covered by disability insurance, and whether you'd retain health insurance with your new schedule). Once you've done your homework, write up a detailed proposal for

your boss. Go ahead and flesh out exactly how your ideal schedule would work. Are you thinking part-time? Flex time? Do you want to telecommute? And what sort of workload could you handle in that amount of time? It may also help to mention who could take on any responsibilities you'll be casting aside, and how you'll train them.

Next, set up a meeting and have a heart-to-heart with the boss. She'll appreciate that you've organized the details in a way that makes the plan easy to implement, upping your chances of getting your way. Talk it out (be ready to compromise) and make a plan. Be sure to get the final agreement in writing (and send a copy to your human resources department) to avoid misunderstandings later on. (Disclaimer: Only you know your boss and your company. We can't promise that she'll go for it.)

> I plan to write a simple, flexible birth plan with the understanding that things may have to change. Why not have something written down so you don't have to think when you're in the moment?
>
> *qmommy*

"Do I really need a birth plan?"
A "birth plan" is really just a way for you to communicate with your partner, doctors, and nurses about delivery-day issues like pain meds, people involved, episiotomies, and cord cutting. The plan can be anything from a simple "I want to avoid interventions if at all possible," or "I'd like you to do whatever you can to keep me from feeling pain" to a full page of desires for labor and childbirth.

If you write up a plan, it's important to talk everything over with your OB to be certain it's realistic and falls in line with hospital policies. After you've cleared your plan with your doctor, make sure there's a copy in your chart and a few copies in the bag you'll take to the hospital. (Have your labor partner hand them out to the labor nurses when you arrive.) If a birth plan is in place, everyone involved in delivery can be reminded of your wishes if decisions need to be made. That way, you can focus on pushing!

It's fine to go without a birth plan, too. Just make sure your labor coach is up to speed on how you feel about different options, since you may not feel much like thinking through big decisions between contractions. And if you do make a written plan, remember that it's nothing but a wish list of basic guidelines. Your (and your babies'!) health and safety come first, and birth plans often change.

"What are the chances of bringing multiples to full term?"
You're about six times as likely to deliver before your due date. Why are so many twins, triplets, and other multiples born early? Think of it this way: Your uterus is a pretty amazing place, but even the womb has its limits. The more baby (plus fluids, plus placenta) in there, the more distended it can become, which means

"do your chances of having
preemies increase with
the number of multiples?"

Most twin pregnancies average about 35 weeks, which means
they're pretty well cooked by the time they're here. (For triplets,
the mark's a little shorter, usually about 33 weeks; quads are 29.)
Although most premature babies receive an excellent prognosis,
it's natural to worry about going early. Experts say you can start
to breathe a little easier past the 32-week mark, since by then the
lungs and other key organs are fully developed. And those who
make it to the 37-week mark are actually considered full term.

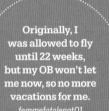

real moms uncensored

on travel...

Originally, I was allowed to fly until 22 weeks, but my OB won't let me now, so no more vacations for me.
femmefatalenat01

I always made sure to get an aisle seat since I had to pee so much!
tarzanswife

I flew three times when I was pregnant. Once I took my shoes off during the flight, and when I tried to put them back on at the end, my feet were too swollen!
sunny1in tucson

We went to Florida when I was about 22 weeks and I was already pretty big, so the flight was uncomfortable. I'd say 20 weeks is the latest I would travel.
home_slice

you have a higher chance of breaking your water, developing preterm contractions, or having your cervix dilate.

"Do I have to have a c-section just because I'm pregnant with multiples, or is there a possibility of delivering vaginally?"

It's true many multiple births are delivered by c-section, but it's certainly possible to deliver multiples vaginally. In fact, about half of twin births are vaginal. That option becomes much less likely with triplets, quads, or pregnancies involving even more babies. But every pregnancy is different. If your doctors think the labor is too difficult, or one or more of the infants is in the breech or compound position, chances are, you'll have to undergo a c-section. If you have a strong preference for a vaginal birth, it's best to talk to your doctor about this in advance so your wishes can be taken into consideration when it comes to delivery day.

"How often do mixed deliveries happen, when one baby is born vaginally and the other one is born by c-section?"

Since twins can be delivered vaginally about half the time, this is the preferred method of delivery for many women. However, it is possible that a problem will occur with the second baby after the first baby is born. In these cases, an emergency c-section may be performed. The result: a "mixed delivery." Luckily, though, this is pretty rare, happening to only 3 to 4 percent of twin births.

"What are the risks my babies face if born prematurely?"

The healthiest place for babies to be until they reach full term is inside Mom's womb, which is why premature birth can result in various complications that make it harder for babies to survive. Some of the more serious complications can include fluid accumulation or bleeding in the brain, trouble breathing, developmental delays, and vision or hearing problems. But before you start worrying too much, it's important to know that not all preemies experience these complications— or any others, for that matter. So, while the risks are certainly higher with preemies, even the tiniest babies can overcome the obstacles associated with preterm birth and grow up to be just as healthy as full-term babies.

"Should I be doing kick counts?"

Kick counts are an easy way to check in on your babies and catch problems early so they can be addressed. There are a lot of different methods for counting your babies' karate chops, so ask your OB for specific suggestions. A common way to do this is to time how long it takes to feel 6 to 10 movements. Pick a time every day to tune in to your tummy and simply count the kicks, swishes, bumps, and jabs. If you

tally between 6 and 10 movements in under an hour, check it off your list until tomorrow. If it takes longer than two hours, or if you notice any big deviations from the norm (like, if it usually takes 15 minutes but now takes 55 minutes), play it safe and give your OB a ring.

Start kick counts as soon as you've hit a point in your pregnancy when you feel your babies squirming on a regular basis (if this doesn't happen by week 26, talk to your doc), and do your kick counts at a time of day when your babies are typically most active, like after dinner or when you lie down in bed at night. If things seem slow, try downing a glass of cold milk—the sugar and temperature should hype the babies up—and lying on your left side, which increases blood flow.

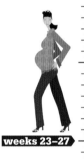

weeks 23–27

"I don't think I've felt the babies kick in a while, and it's worrying me. How can I make them kick?"

After 26 weeks, you should be feeling regular daily fetal movements. This works a little differently for everyone, but generally you'll notice those little ones wriggling around in there.

If you haven't felt your little ones kick in a bit and you miss those jabs, lie on your side (to increase blood flow to the babies), drink some juice or eat something, and count your fetal movements. Each fetus should move about 6 to 10 times an hour—any roll, swish, jab, or other fetal movement counts. (Worried about how you'll know which baby is kicking? Close your eyes and focus; you'll likely be able to tell your babies' movements apart. If you can't, talk to your doctor about how to distinguish between them.) If you don't feel enough kicks when you do your counts, get in touch with your OB.

❚ is it normal?

"I have terrible gas! What's going on…and what can I do?"

At least the gas is for a good cause: The hormone progesterone is relaxing smooth muscles in your gastrointestinal tract to make your gut work slower, giving your body more time to snatch up nutrients from your food and take them to your babies. Unfortunately, a slower gut can translate into some serious belches and toots. Soon your growing uterus will start pushing up on your stomach and down on your rectum, too, compounding the problem. To help relieve the pressure, eat small, regular meals and stay away from foods that tend to give you gas. You know the culprits: fried stuff, dairy, beans, dried fruit, brussels sprouts, cabbage, and so on. Eating and drinking slowly will also keep you from swallowing excess air. Taking a yoga class can help settle things down too. And ward off constipation (a big gas-inducer) with plenty of liquids and high-fiber foods.

"I'm on my feet a ton at work. What can I do to ease the foot and back pain?"

Between your shifting center of balance, all that extra weight, and loosening ligaments, it's no wonder that you're aching. If you can't get off your feet (ask for breaks and prop up your tootsies when you can!), be sure to wear comfy shoes with good support, and try adding a gel insole—they make them for heels now too! Speaking of heels, they aren't a total no-no. Retire your stilettos, but keep out the kitten heels—1½- to 2-inch heels may actually provide extra support for your back. If you start to have a lot of trouble with swelling, consider support hose, which can keep the blood from pooling in your feet. You might also benefit from a pregnancy support belt, especially as you grow even larger. It can seriously ease the stress on your back. (Bonus: Some moms say it takes a load off their bladder too!) Also, make a special effort to maintain good posture—your back (make that your whole body) will thank you.

"I just realized I have hemorrhoids! What can I do about them?"

You've got extra blood flowing through your veins right now, and it can sometimes pool up in the parts of your body most affected by gravity (such as, yes, the rectum). The result is swollen, itchy varicose veins, and when these come where the sun don't shine, they're called hemorrhoids. Your growing uterus is also adding pressure to the region, making it prone to swelling.

Talk to your OB about creams and suppositories that you can use to ease the pain,

"what's a 'normal' weight for a multiple?"

About half of all twins weigh at least 5½ pounds at birth. (Below 5½ pounds, or 2,500 grams, is considered a low birth weight, with a higher potential for complications.) In comparison, the average singleton weighs 7 pounds, but it's not that she's comparatively bigger, it's because on average she's hanging out in utero for another five weeks. That said, it's not unusual for some women to deliver twins that each weigh around 7 pounds if the pregnancy lasts until week 37 (just think how much better you'd feel when you were done carrying that load around). The average triplet weighs 4 pounds at birth, and the average quad 3 pounds. While they might have to spend a few days in the NICU putting on some weight, the good news is, many preemies are considered "feeders and growers," which means they'll soon catch up to their peers. Keep a record of your babies' every move throughout your pregnancy.

weeks 23–27

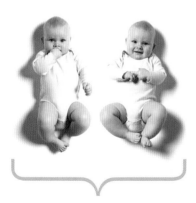

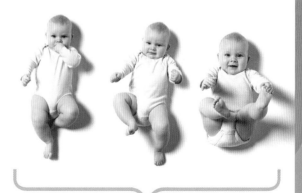

average twin birth weight:
5½ pounds

average triplet birth weight:
4 pounds

experiment with hot or cold packs, or try witch hazel pads and sitz baths (soaking the area in a little hot water). Constipation (and the straining it leads to) may also be the culprit, so make an extra effort to stay hydrated and eat lots of fiber. If you still can't get regular, ask your doctor which stool softeners are safe. Excess weight can make hemorrhoids worse, so try to stay within your doctor's recommended guidelines, and don't forget to exercise— even if it's not so comfortable right now. When you get moving, you'll ease the pressure on the veins in your pelvic area. (It'll help the constipation too.) And finally, keep up your Kegels (see page 88)—they can help increase circulation to the area.

"I'm waking up with awful leg cramps! How can I keep from getting them?"
Leg cramps are common as you enter the last months of pregnancy. Doctors aren't sure why, but they suspect it has something to do with changes in circulation, the extra weight you're carrying, or babies pressing on nerves and blood vessels. Whatever the reason, they can be a serious pain.

To keep cramps at bay, try stretching and massaging your calves before bed and in the morning, and adding bananas to your diet (some experts think the potassium might help). If you find yourself stretching out your legs when you lie in bed, don't point your toes! (Chances are, they'll get stuck there.) When the cramps come on, enlist your partner to grab your leg and flex

your feet, or stand and do a lunge beside the bed. Once the pain eases up a little, walking around for a few minutes can help relax the muscle.

"My boobs are totally killing me! Why, and when will it end?"
Breast tenderness is one of the first signs of pregnancy, and while it usually fades by the end of the first trimester, it can last longer for some women. We've heard of moms-to-be well into their second trimester describe the feeling "like someone put jumper cables on my nipples every time a cool breeze goes by." Your best defense: a good supportive bra (some women even like to wear a pregnancy sleep bra at night), along with liberal amounts of a heavy balm to prevent chafing. See more on bras on page 34.

is it safe?

"What can my babies hear? Do I need to stay away from loud noise?"
Those tiny inner ears have been forming since month 4, but now they're becoming well developed. Go ahead and sing, chat, read, and play your favorite tunes for your mini-me. Studies show that, while lots of sounds are filtered out by the uterine wall and amniotic fluid, babies are able to hear, respond to, and remember sounds from their time in the womb. It's the lower-frequency noises that make it through, so go heavy on the bass. As

for volume, you should be fine taking in a concert or sitting by a horde of screaming football fans—just be ready for the babies to react to all the hoopla, especially during the last trimester. The jury's still out on whether frequent loud noises are truly safe. If you work in an especially noisy place (we're talking about loud machinery here, not your annoying cube mates), talk with your OB about what you can do.

"Is it okay for the babies to sleep in the same crib?"

Yes! In fact, many pediatricians encourage it. You know how your bed seems empty when your partner is out of town? Think about how you'd feel if the two of you were together there 24 hours a day, for 35 weeks or more, then suddenly pulled apart. For twins, having each other close by is comforting, since they've been together since the get-go. So go ahead and let them sleep in the same crib. It's totally safe, especially in the first few weeks, when they're tightly swaddled and hardly move around. Once they start wiggling more and risk bumping each other, try a crib divider, which slips from side rail to side rail and splits the crib into two so each infant has his or her own space. Most models have Velcro attachments that go around the slats to stay in place. You can keep the divider for a few months, until the babies get big enough to need their own, separate cribs.

"I'm sick of walking. What are some fun ways to get my exercise in while I'm pregnant?"

Check with your doctor before starting a new routine, but thirty minutes of exercise a day (with your OB's approval) can lower your risk of complications like diabetes and pre-eclampsia. Plus, it's associated with shorter labors and quicker recoveries—pretty good incentives, if you ask us. No matter what new exercise you try, make sure to tell the instructor you're pregnant so she can modify moves as necessary. And pay close attention to how you feel.

SWIMMING

WHY IT'S GOOD The pool lets you feel weightless for a change, taking a load off joints and compressed organs while you work a wide range of muscle groups.

WHAT TO TRY Gentle laps or a basic water aerobics class

YOGA

WHY IT'S GOOD Not only is yoga great for your body, but you'll learn breathing and relaxation techniques that can be a big help during labor, and positions to try if you'll be going sans epidural.

WHAT TO TRY Prenatal yoga or a basic, level-one class

PILATES

WHY IT'S GOOD Since it focuses on your core, Pilates can improve your posture, prevent backaches, and even help when it's time for you to push.

WHAT TO TRY Prenatal mat classes or a basic mat class

weeks 23–27

BELLY DANCING

WHY IT'S GOOD The traditional Middle Eastern dance was used in ancient times to help women get ready for childbirth, soothing their babies and preparing their bodies for delivery.

WHAT TO TRY Any class you can find! Or a good DVD

the day-to-day

"When do we need to start figuring out what to do about child care?"

Last week. Just kidding (sort of)—the answer to this one depends on where you live and what kind of care you're looking for. If you're shooting for a day-care facility (stimulating environment, interaction with other kids), you'll probably need to apply pronto. Day cares in major cities can have waiting lists out the wazoo (as in 9 to 12 months or more). Prefer an in-home nanny (personal attention, more flexible schedules, higher cost)? Put your feelers out for recommendations, but you should be okay holding off on interviews until your babies are around to help pick their match.

"What are Kegels? How do I do them?"

Kegels are exercises that help strengthen the muscles on your pelvic floor, which support your uterus, bladder, and bowel. What's the point? Do these, and you'll be less likely to pee your pants when babies begin pressing on your bladder in the third trimester. Kegels will help with similar problems postdelivery too. Plus, one 2004 study even showed that they can shorten the second phase of labor (the pushing part). Add in the fact that Kegels are known to help out in the bedroom (they make it easier to orgasm), and this is one exercise you don't want to slack on.

There are different ways to do a Kegel, and some experts think it's best to mix it up. First, find the right muscles by attempting to stop your urine midstream a couple of times. Feel the muscles that you use? Those are the Kegels. (Don't routinely practice your Kegels while you tinkle, though. It can actually weaken the muscles.) Now imagine smoothly drawing those pelvic floor muscles up like an elevator. Hold at the top for a count of 10; then slowly lower muscles to the starting position. Repeat 10 times. For some variation, quickly contract and release the muscles 10 times in a row. Take a break, and then repeat the exercise 10 more times.

"Should I take a Lamaze class?"

Sure, why not? Used by one-fourth of all mothers, Lamaze is by far the most popular childbirth method. You'll learn simple, natural strategies like rhythmic breathing, hydrotherapy, massage, position changes, and walking to use during delivery. Your labor partner will also learn how to encourage and support you. The classes (at least 12 hours overall) include a wide range of info on what to expect during and after delivery, possible complications, how to be an active participant and effectively communicate with hospital staff, and tips for breastfeeding and interacting once baby comes. Contrary to what you may have heard, Lamaze is not anti-pain meds; all of your options will be covered during class. Interested in other childbirth methods? You might want to check out Bradley, Alexander, or Hypnobirthing.

"So many kinds of strollers! Which to choose?"

Obviously, you'll need a multiples stroller to carry all your babies. Here's the scoop on which kind is best for you:

Most parents definitely favor side-by-side strollers because they mean both kids have the same view and, in most cases, both seats can fully recline. They're also usually a little less bulky. The disadvantage is that these wide-bodies can be harder to maneuver through tight spaces, and in some cases they won't squeeze through a doorway.

Tandem (front/back) strollers ensure a lot more room to move around (and get a lot fewer dirty looks if you're strolling on a crowded sidewalk or in a store with lots of racks or shelves!). Some models also accommodate two infant car seats, so you can go straight to the tandem and skip the snap-and-go. On the not-so-good side: Tandems are usually heavier, and typically only the back seat can recline fully. Plus, there's bound to be an unhappy customer if one gets the blocked rear view.

Jogging strollers are for parents who dream of working off some pregnancy weight with regular power walks or runs, and they're a necessity if you want to avoid completely killing your back while doing so. If you're a walker, consider getting one with a front wheel that swivels, which is a bit easier to handle when it comes to making turns. If you're more of a runner, consider a model with a fixed front wheel, which will track straighter and handle bumps better.

If you have quads or more, your stroller options are limited. It's very difficult to find all-terrain or jogger strollers for triplets or more (but do you really want to push four or more kids while you run?), but if you're expecting twins or triplets, you have tons of jogger options.

If you're looking for something that you can use until your babies hit toddlerhood, try a convertible stroller. There are plenty of models available for multiples. You can find descriptions and real mom reviews of the latest options at TheBump.com/gear.

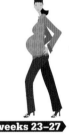

weeks 23–27

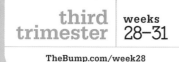

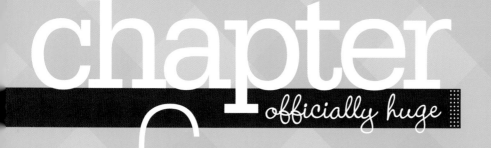

chapter five

officially huge

you've made it to the third trimester! The end is in sight—just a few weeks away—and you're probably still feeling semi-good, though some fatigue may be sneaking back in, you're running to the bathroom again, and it's getting tougher to tie your shoes. This is a good time to start making serious plans for your new life with your babies (finding a pediatrician, stocking up on bottles, familiarizing yourself with the car seats, trying not to freak out). You're probably starting to think about the reality of labor and delivery too. Yes, your babies are going to eventually come out. And if you think your belly is ginormous now, just wait—it's still got a long way to go!

your to-do list

- Find a pediatrician

- Take a tour of the maternity ward

- Preregister with the hospital

- Sign up for a breastfeeding class

Get our complete pediatrician checklist at Thebump.com/pedi

what you're in for...

66

bed rest

ouch!

my boobs just started leaking.

WHAT DOES IT MEAN IF I MEASURE BIG?

I have to pee all the time.

I'm such a klutz.

I'm still feeling so tired.

MY FEET ARE EVEN MORE SWOLLEN!

insanely itchy belly and boobs! 99

on your mind...

▌ at the ob's office

"What does it mean if I'm measuring too small or too big at the doctor's office?"

When you visit your OB after 20 weeks, she may measure the distance from your pubic bone to the top of your uterus, which is known as the fundal height. Moms expecting singletons are measured regularly, but many docs won't even measure women pregnant with multiples. Unfortunately, when you're having twins or more, it's more difficult to assess "average" fundal height. However, as long as you are gaining weight consistently and sufficiently and your fundal height is growing steadily, your doc will likely be satisfied.

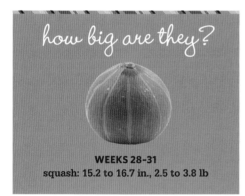

how big are they?

WEEKS 28–31
squash: 15.2 to 16.7 in., 2.5 to 3.8 lb

If your OB does measure you and says that you are too big or too small, she will schedule you for an ultrasound to check things out.

POSSIBLE REASONS FOR MEASURING LARGE:

- You simply have big, healthy babies
- Your due date is wrong
- You have gestational diabetes

POSSIBLE REASONS FOR MEASURING SMALL:

- Your babies are small
- Your due date is wrong

"What does going on bed rest really mean?"

Being told to go on bed rest can be a dreaded order, but it doesn't have to mean your life is totally on hold. The definition of bed rest isn't the same for every expectant mother, and the key is to find out from your doctor what your specific limitations are. Some bed rest orders may be very strict, meaning your doctor doesn't want you to sit on the couch or get up to grab a quick bite or even shower. But for others, bed rest has a broader definition, so it may be safe to be up for short periods of time or even to drive to the doctor's office. Make sure to talk with your OB about what, specifically, you can and can't do while on bed rest, so you know just how active you're allowed to be. It's also a good idea to find out if there's a particular position you should be lying in while resting that's best for your babies' health.

weeks 28–31 ▶

"What are things I can do to keep babies from coming too early?"

Your pregnancy time line is a little different from that of moms expecting singletons; you'll likely be giving birth before 40 weeks. But you don't want them to come too early since low birth weight is a concern.

Twins should ideally be born at 38 weeks, triplets between 36 and 37 weeks, and quads at 36 weeks.

While you can't prevent preterm labor, you can lower the risk. Here's how:

- Start prenatal care ASAP and keep all of your OB appointments
- Maintain a healthy pregnancy weight and eat enough calories derived from the nutrients recommended to you (see page 59)
- Drink lots of water
- Don't smoke or use drugs
- Call your doctor anytime you feel sick
- Don't stress

Be vigilant for signs of preterm labor. To protect yourself and your babies, get familiar with preterm labor symptoms, like regular or severe contractions. Keep on the lookout for contractions that occur four or more times in an hour, lower back pain, pelvic pressure, vaginal discharge tinged with blood, menstrual-like cramps, or diarrhea. Talk to your doctor about how to recognize preterm labor, and if you experience any of those symptoms, call the doctor immediately—you may be able to convince those babies to stay put with your OB's help. Never, ever feel shy about calling your doctor if you're worried.

❚ in your head

"If I fall, will it hurt the babies?"

The combo of a shifting center of balance and ligament-loosening hormones swimming around can definitely make you clumsy. First off, you can prevent falls by wearing comfortable shoes with nonskid soles (this is NOT the time for 4-inch heels), holding on to railings on the stairs, avoiding slick surfaces, and being extra-careful in general. If you do happen to suffer a fall, don't panic. Your babies are very well padded in their fluid-filled home, and aren't likely to be hurt at all. Do call your OB, though—she might want to check out the babies' heartbeats, just to make sure all is well.

"I just realized that these babies actually have to come OUT. I'm starting to panic!"

First, know that it's completely normal to be nervous. If you start feeling overwhelmed, it might help to think of all the women through-out history who gave birth before you (and how many didn't enjoy the luxury of a hospital room and an OB!). Every single person in the world was born, and most of them came out of a vagina. That means there is a darn good chance you'll get through this just fine. If that rationale doesn't calm you, try finding something that does, like yoga, meditation, talking it out with a trusted friend, or reading about other moms' experiences.

"Be honest—what exactly will a vaginal birth do to my vagina?"

Yes, pushing human beings out of such a small opening is scary to every one of us. Don't freak, though. Your body is amazing, and it's made to go through this. Here's the real-life scoop on what your vagina is in for. (If you don't want to know, don't read on.)

Will your vagina be exactly the same as it was before? No—probably not. Most couples

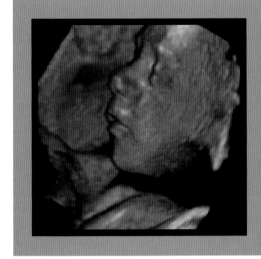

what babies are up to

- kicking extra hard and often
- packing on the fat layer
- brains are growing a bunch
- lungs begin to function
- lanugo starts to disappear
- have eyebrows and eyelashes
- have smooth, pink skin
- eyes have color (they might change after delivery)

report some degree of noticeable change . . . but they also tend to say it isn't so bad. Your vagina will do some serious stretching as the babies slides out, and you will be swollen and bruised for a while. As you recover during the next couple of weeks, your vagina will gradually shrink back down (though maybe not all the way). To help regain muscle tone and tighten things up, keep up your Kegels, especially in the weeks following delivery. These exercises will also help to keep you from leaking urine after you deliver (pretty common after the stresses of childbirth) as well as after menopause.

Your vagina may tear during delivery, or you might have an episiotomy (the doctor could make a cut to enlarge the opening). In either case, you'll likely be stitched up and will heal in 6 weeks or so. Your perineum (the skin between your vagina and rectum)

could look noticeably different, depending on the degree of tearing and the skill of the person who did the stitching. If there's a difference, it will most likely be subtle. You may also be left with a bit of scar tissue, which can be uncomfortable during your first attempts at postpartum sex. Each woman's experience is different, but you should feel back to normal (or close to it, at least) after a few (or a few dozen) rolls in the hay. One more temporary vaginal alteration: You'll probably be really dry, especially if you're breastfeeding. Lube is your friend.

weeks 28–31

"Should I choose a pediatrician who specializes in multiples?"

There's a lot that needs to get done during the time you're pregnant with multiples, so don't be upset when I add one more thing to the list: Find a pediatrician who's right for your family! It's great to find a pediatrician who is familiar with treating multiples, and it's key to choose a doctor who understands the developmental issues that are often associated with prematurity, but the important part is finding a doctor whom you feel comfortable with. Do some research before your babies are born, so you know exactly where to take them for their first doctor's visit. While your multiples pregnancy should be treated very differently from a singleton pregnancy, the same isn't necessarily true once your babies are out of the womb.

is it normal?

"Ahh! I have to pee all the time again. How can I cut down on bathroom trips?"

Between the masses of extra blood in your body (meaning more fluids running through your kidneys) and the pressure created by your ever-expanding (shall we say giant?) uterus, it's no wonder you're always in the loo. You won't find complete relief until the babies arrive, but here are three tips for spending a little less time on the toilet.

GET IT ALL OUT Make an effort to empty your bladder completely every time you pee. Lean forward to add a little bit of pressure to your bladder and get all the urine out. Bonus: This also helps prevent UTIs.

DRINK THE RIGHT STUFF Stay away from coffee, tea, and alcohol, all of which can keep you running to the ladies' room. (You should be steering clear of alcohol and more than two servings of caffeine daily anyway, of course.)

EASE UP IN THE EVENING Curbing your liquids in the hours before bedtime might make your nightly bathroom runs less frequent. If you go this route, just be sure to get plenty of fluids in the daytime—hydration is extra important as you move toward the big day.

delivery countdown

"How do I preregister with the hospital? (And why do I have to?)"

Preregistering will take care of your basic admission paperwork so your file is all ready to go on delivery day. If your hospital offers preregistration, it can save you some hassle—and maybe even get you into a room faster—when your babies finally decide to make an appearance. Check with your hospital to find out what you need to do. Often, it's as simple as filling out a single form, and you may be able to do it over the telephone or online. It usually takes a few minutes, and can save you from digging for your insurance card—and having to think— once you're in active labor.

"Are there exercises I can do that will make giving birth easier?"

Giving birth probably won't be "easy" no matter what you do, but it certainly does involve muscles, breathing, and endurance. Flexibility helps too—and all of these are things you can work on to help your body

"what should I pack in my hospital bag?"

It's a good idea to have your bag ready by around week 32. Here's what should be in it:

- Pairs of warm nonskid socks that can get ruined
- Pajamas
- Your own pillow and/or pillowcase (obviously, the hospital will provide these, but your own may help you feel comfortable)
- A warm robe or cardigan sweater (maternity wards can be really cold, so be prepared)
- 3 maternity bras— no underwire— and nursing pads (whether or not you plan to nurse)
- Personal-hygiene items, like a toothbrush, toothpaste, moisturizer, and deodorant

- Lip balm (hospitals are very dry)
- Going-home clothes (in maternity sizes; just because the babies came out doesn't mean your old body will be back yet) and flat shoes
- Headband or ponytail holders
- Glasses and/or contacts, if you wear them
- Makeup (so you can look good in those first photos!)
- Sanitary napkins (the hospital will provide these, but you may prefer your own)
- Maternity underwear that can get ruined; you'll get some disposal pairs at the hospital—some women find them

very handy and others think they're gross, so bring your own just to be safe
- iPod or music for the delivery room
- Earplugs (if you want to block out the surrounding noise and be Zen)
- Receiving blankets to swaddle the babies
- Going-home outfits for your babies
- Warm baby blankets (for the ride home)
- Insurance info, hospital forms, and birth plan (if you have one)
- Sugar-free hard candy or lozenges to keep your mouth moist during labor (candy with sugar will make you thirsty)

- Pen and paper
- Very light reading (think magazines and newspapers)
- Diaper bag
- Car seats (one for each child)
- Camera, film or extra memory card, battery or charger
- Lots of change for the vending machines and nonperishable snacks (you'll probably be hungry after the births, and the hospital cafeteria could be closed)
- Cell phone and charger, contact list (so you can call people after the births), and prepaid calling card (if the hospital doesn't allow cell phones)

weeks 28–31

what to skip

Jewelry

Lots of cash

Breast pump

Laptop (your colleagues are not expecting that e-mail; give work a rest!)

Diapers (the hospital will provide them)

Baby book (you won't have time or energy to write)

prepare for the hard work of labor. Here are a few exercises to try (just be sure to get the all-clear from your OB first).

HIP OPENERS Sit on the floor with the soles of your feet pressed together and your knees open wide in a diamond shape. Use your elbows to open the hips further, and hold for 30 to 60 seconds. Opening your hips helps to make room for babies' arrival.

AB CLENCHES You'll definitely need your abs when it's time to start pushing. (Yes, they might be stretched out, but they're still there.) Traditional crunches aren't practical, though—you shouldn't lie on your back, and improper form could cause your abs to tear. Instead, sit or stand up straight and focus on pulling your navel back toward your spine. Hold it there for a few breaths and release. Like Kegels, you can do these just about anywhere. Try to hold this pose as often as possible to protect and condition your abs.

MODERATE CARDIO Stay active by walking, swimming, or taking a prenatal workout class. You'll appreciate the lung capacity and heart conditioning when it comes time to breathe through contractions.

"I overheard someone at the OB talking about a VBAC. What is that?"

It stands for "vaginal birth after cesarean." Not long ago, one c-section meant you were destined to have a cesarean for every child, but now 60 to 80 percent of women who've had a c-section can give birth to future children the old-fashioned way. If you had a c-section for one child,

bring up the idea of VBAC with your OB. Chances are, you'll be able to deliver vaginally this time around.

"How early should I expect to go into labor?"

Twins tend to arrive sooner than singleton babies. While single babies develop for an average of 39 weeks, twins tend to appear around 35 weeks. (Triplets often arrive even sooner, by about 32 weeks; and quadruplets cook for an average of about 29 weeks.)

"If I am having twins, will I definitely need to have a c-section?"

Not necessarily. It depends on your babies' size and position. If they are both head-down, then you can deliver vaginally, and many twin moms do. No matter what, you'll need to deliver in a hospital, and you should find an OB skilled in twin deliveries to help ensure all goes well. (More babies mean a higher risk of complications.)

When you arrive at the hospital, you'll probably have an ultrasound to confirm that your babies are head-down and ready to go. Then you'll labor just like a singleton mom. When it's time for delivery, you'll probably be wheeled into an operating room instead of a regular delivery room. This is in case one or both twins wind up needing an emergency c-section. (Sometimes the first twin can be born vaginally but the second one has to come by cesarean.) After your first twin arrives, your OB will check on your second to see if he's well positioned for delivery. If so, the

checklist

"what questions should I ask when I tour the hospital?"

Some Qs, like "What will my room look like?" and "Where should we park?" will likely be answered without your asking, but you should come armed with anything (and everything) else you've been wondering. Here are some questions to get you started:

○ Can I preregister a couple of weeks in advance? Can I do it online? (Getting some legal hoopla out of the way can be very freeing.)

○ When we arrive, do we need to check in at the front desk first, or can I waddle straight to the maternity ward?

○ What are the policies on cameras and video cameras? (Also, ask about these policies in the OR, because multiples—even when delivered vaginally—are often birthed in an OR, which may have very stringent rules about recording devices.)

○ Are cell phones allowed?

○ How many people are allowed in the delivery room?

○ What if I go in for a c-section? Can someone come with me?

○ Can my partner stay the night?

○ What levels of NICU care are available? If my babies need intensive care, will they have to be transported to another hospital? How far away, and how will they get there?

○ How soon after giving birth can I try to breastfeed?

○ Can I get a private room? Will my insurance cover it?

○ Will my babies be able to stay in my room throughout my stay at the hospital?

○ Will the nursing staff look after my babies if I need a break? How does that process work?

○ What sort of breastfeeding support is offered? How does it work?

○ Where and when are my other children allowed to be with me?

weeks 28–31

car seat

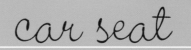

head support Look for special insert to support the infant's wobbly head. Only use one that comes with the seat.

harness A five-point harness is a must. Look for straps that are easy to adjust and a buckle that's not tricky to unlatch.

insert If your baby is under 5 lbs, you'll need to add an insert to your infant car seat.

comfort Do the material and padding feel soft and snuggly? This may sound like a luxury, but trust us —anything that helps soothe babies is essential those first few months.

energy-absorbing foam During an accident, this is what keeps the baby safe and protected from impact.

side protection Deep side walls and adequate barriers around the head protect the baby from a side-impact accident.

blankets Jackets can affect the way the baby sits in the car seat and impact how it performs, so it's better to dress the baby normally, then keep him warm with blankets.

registration Register your car seat so you'll be notified of any recalls or updates.

expiration date Yes, car seats have them. Normal life span is about six years.

you'll also see

MIRRORS AND TOYS Though these may seem like great ways to keep babies distracted and calm during a car ride, they have the potential of turning into hazardous flying objects during a car accident. Even seemingly innocuous toys that clip onto the car seat can be a problem, as they may affect the way it performs.

OB may break your water to encourage baby number two to move along. The contractions will restart soon (or you'll get some Pitocin to help them along), and you can then start pushing, the same way as before.

"Will I have to give birth at a special hospital for high-risk pregnancies?"
It depends on the amount—and type—of pregnancy. If you're carrying fraternal twins or identicals who have their own space in the womb, a general OB working in your local hospital can be perfectly capable of welcoming them into the world. But for triplets or higher-order multiples, and for identicals who are buddying up in a single sac or sharing a placenta, you'll be better off delivering at a hospital that can offer a bigger safety net in case you need it, since the chances of complications are significantly higher.

"Will my birth classes be different? When should I start taking them?"
Babies are babies, so many of the concepts covered in child-prep classes (changing diapers, learning to swaddle, breastfeeding) apply across the board, no matter how many you're carrying. But there are distinct differences between singles and multiples. For one, you're more likely to go into premature labor, so it's important to be on the lookout for signs of early labor (pelvic pressure, low back pain, increased vaginal discharge, a change in the amount of "false labor" pains). And since the logistics of coping with twins or more can be overwhelming, you might find it helpful to take a class that's devoted to caring for multiples. As for timing, since you can expect to go a little early, it's probably not too soon to start taking classes in your second trimester.

▌the day-to-day
"How do I find a pediatrician?"
Good old-fashioned word of mouth is the best way to find a great doctor. Can't think of whom to ask? You can also corner new moms (in a nice way) for advice as they're picking up their tots from the nursery at church or shopping at a local baby store. They've been in your shoes, so chances are good they'll be happy to help. (Your pregnant belly will keep you from looking too creepy.) Online reviews can be helpful as well, as can moms on your local online message boards.

weeks 28–31 ▶

Log on to your insurance company's website (or give them a call) to access a list of local doctors who are covered by your plan. Once you've narrowed it down to a couple of candidates, begin making phone calls and setting up consultations (don't worry, these are usually free). A quick round of interviews will help you to find a great match. And remember not to stress too much: You can switch doctors at any time. This decision isn't permanent.

breastfeeding 411

"What are the benefits of breastfeeding?"

Breast milk contains the perfect mix of enzymes and antibodies, making breastfed babies less likely to have ear infections, colds, diarrhea, respiratory problems, allergies, and stomach bugs. Plus, nursing decreases future risk of obesity, diabetes, inflammatory bowel disease, childhood leukemia, and other forms of cancer.

There are perks for you too. It won't cost you a penny, requires no prep, is always wherever you are, and it comes out at the perfect temperature. It also can help you lose weight, heal more quickly down below, and has been linked to decreased breast cancer and uterine cancer.

"Will I be able to breastfeed multiples?"

Even if you deliver early, your body will be ready to start producing milk soon after you give birth. In fact, in preterm infants, the mother's milk is actually higher in protein and other nutrients that can strengthen babies' immune systems and help them gain weight. Many mothers of multiples become milk-making machines, but keep in mind that it can be challenging for any new mom to get even one newborn to feed, let alone two or more. Don't get discouraged—it takes time and practice to get your babies to latch on. In the meantime, keep your production up by pumping, and don't be shy about asking a lactation consultant for assistance.

real moms uncensored on **breastfeeding...**

I did pump in the beginning to try to help my milk come in faster, and to get a small freezer stash. I also pumped when I was sending them to day care for a few hours, a few days a week, so I could get some rest. *kaitley44*

Hang in there! The first 8 weeks or so were so hard, but now it is wonderful. Lactation consultants really helped me a lot. *jalaiaa*

I BF my twins and I'm doing it tandem, so I don't switch sides in the middle of the feed. I just let them stay on the same side and then make sure to rotate each baby to the other side at the next feed. Then I pump with a hospital-grade pump after every session to get enough milk for each twin for nighttime feedings. *nygrl79*

checklist

"what do I ask when I interview the pediatrician?"

Most important, you want to get a general feel for whether the doctor's personality, views, and communication style mesh with yours. You'll probably have only about 10 minutes to test the vibe, so ask questions that are most important to you first. Here are some to consider:

- How long have you been practicing?
- Do you have any subspecialties?
- What are your hours?
- Do you offer same-day sick appointments? How far in advance do well appointments need to be scheduled?
- What if one of my babies get sick when the office is closed?
- Is this a solo or group practice? If it's solo, who covers when you are gone? If it's a group, how often will we see you, and how often will we see others?
- Do you have separate sick and well waiting rooms?

- Do you respond to questions by e-mail? If I leave a message, how long does it usually take you to return the call?
- Will your initial meeting with my babies be at the hospital or the first checkup? What is your schedule for well-baby checkups?
- Will you discuss general growth and issues like discipline and social development?
- What are your views on . . . bottle-feeding? Circumcision? Parenting techniques? Getting babies to sleep? Alternative medicine? Antibiotics? Immunizations?
- What hospitals do you work with?

- Do you take my insurance? Is there an extra charge for . . . advice calls during the day? Advice calls after hours? Medication refills? Filling out forms? Will any other fees apply?
- What are your policies for insurance claims, lab policies, payments, and billing?
- What tests are handled in the office and what is done elsewhere? Where?
- Are you experienced in working with multiples? How many sets of multiples do you treat?
- Do you have experience working with babies who are preterm?

weeks 28–31

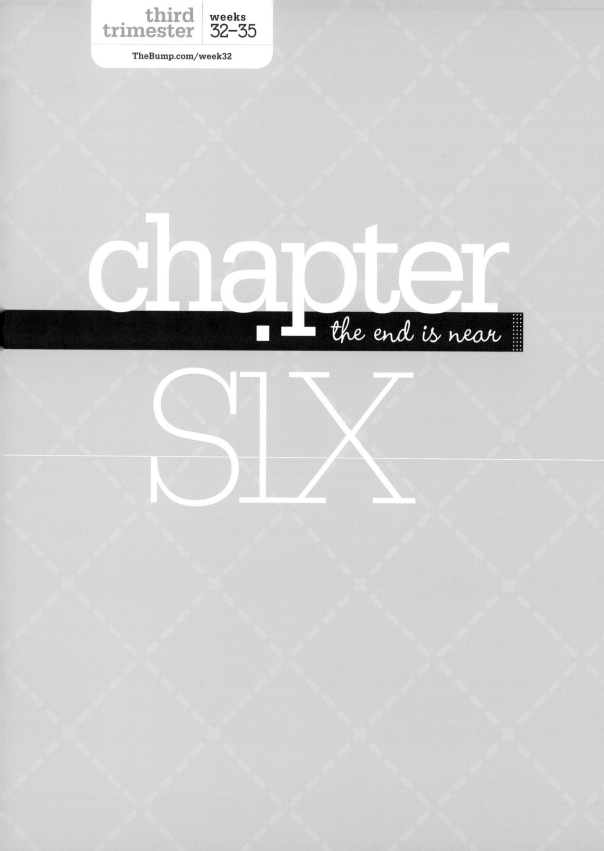

chapter

the end is near

six

tick tock—your babies will be here soon!

Your OB will probably start scheduling your appointments every week at this point. Sure, you're falling asleep in meetings and wetting yourself pretty much whenever you sneeze, but who cares? You're about to be a mom! While babies kick you in the ribs in the middle of the night, you're trying to come up with the perfect middle names. And wondering if you really need special infant-laundry detergent. And how on earth you'll baby-proof an entire house. And if you'll ever have time to cook dinner again. And whether you're really the cloth diaper type. Oh, the list goes on and on!

your to-do list

- Have baby shower
- Pack your hospital bag
- Do some initial baby-proofing
- Cook a few meals to freeze

▸ Download our hospital bag checklist at TheBump.com/bag

what you're in for...

"I CAN'T BELIEVE MY BELLY WILL GET BIGGER THAN THIS!

Is this heavy discharge normal?

UGH... THE PRESSURE

difficult to breathe.

OMG—I JUST PEED WHEN I SNEEZED.

MY BELLY BUTTON POPPED.

ouch!

I'm obsessed with labor.

I'm sooo tired.

My feet barely fit in my shoes."

on your mind...

▌ at the ob's office

"Will the doctor estimate my babies' delivery weight? How?"

Your OB may or may not venture a ballpark guess of your babies' sizes. If she does throw out a number, don't expect it to be spot-on. It's just a guesstimate, based on how big your uterus feels, how you're measuring, and your own stature. That said, many moms report being surprised by their doc's accurate guess!

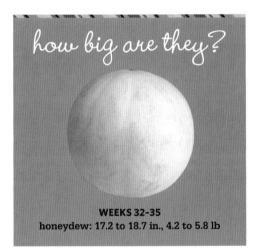

how big are they?

WEEKS 32–35
honeydew: 17.2 to 18.7 in., 4.2 to 5.8 lb

"What is the GBS test?"

For the Group B Strep (GBS) test, your OB will take a quick swab of your vagina and rectum and send the samples to a lab to check for bacteria called group B streptococcus. One in four pregnant women carries GBS, even though most never experience symptoms. If you do have the GBS bacteria floating

around—usually in the reproductive, digestive, or urinary tract—it can be passed to your babies during labor and delivery, and although very few babies contract this infection, those who do can suffer serious disorders or disabilities. If you test positive for GBS, you'll be treated with antibiotics during labor to keep your little ones in the clear.

If you're planning a c-section, antibiotics may not be necessary because babies are typically exposed to GBS during vaginal labor. However, even if you've already scheduled your cesarean, you still need to be tested, in the event that you go into preterm labor. Every pregnant woman should be tested for GBS, so talk to your OB about it. The test should be administered at approximately 35 to 37 weeks for multiples.

▌ in your head

"How can I be sure the babies will fit?"

While it seems like a tight squeeze, you aren't likely to have babies that are larger than your body can handle. Biology just doesn't work that way. Generally speaking, if you're a tiny person, your babies will end up on the small side too. Plus, your tissues have an incredible ability to stretch—and as long as your babies can make it through the smallest part of your pelvic bones, you're golden. To help out, the bones of your babies' skulls don't harden and fuse together until after delivery, allowing

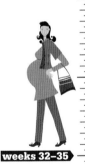

weeks 32–35 ▶

for some squeezing and making your babies' exits a little more streamlined.

"I've been put on bed rest! How do I keep from going insane with worry?"

First, the logistics. Decide where you'd like to set up camp (your bed? the couch?), and have your partner, mom, or friend create a cozy, full-service nest for you. Stock it with a phone, plenty of reading material, paper and pencil, a TV with remote, lots of drinks and snacks (get a cooler for the perishable stuff), and a laptop with Internet access. Some moms like to alternate between mindless entertainment (Sudoku, daytime soaps) and baby preparations (pediatrician hunting, online shopping, making to-do lists for their partner). If your OB says it's okay, a little light exercise—like leg lifts—can get your blood flowing and keep you from feeling too sluggish. As for your emotions, it's normal to feel angry and worried when your pregnancy doesn't go according to plan. Share your feelings with your mate, a trusted friend, or connect with other moms-to-be who are also on bed rest—look for them in online mommy groups.

"Will my babies be breech?"

In the weeks before delivery, most babies shift in the womb so their heads are presenting downward, toward the birth canal. This is the ideal presentation for labor and vaginal birth. However, if one or more of your babies is presenting so the bottom or feet are facing the birth canal, this means she is (or they are) breech. There are three ways a baby could be breech:

COMPLETE BREECH When the baby's bum is down and the legs are folded at the knees.

FOOTLING BREECH When the feet are presenting down.

FRANK BREECH When the bottom is down and the legs stick straight up with the feet at the baby's head.

This is less important for those of you who are expecting triplets or more, because you will probably deliver your babies via c-section, so their presentation doesn't matter as much. But if you're expecting twins and you plan on delivering vaginally, your doctor will evaluate how your babies are presenting before their birth. Unfortunately, multiple babies are more likely to be breech because there is less room in your uterus. Sometimes, though, once the first baby comes out, the second baby will flip into the proper presentation. There is no way to prevent a breech baby; in fact, it's not always known why this occurs, but a few factors that may contribute are:

- Your uterus has too much or too little amniotic fluid
- You've been pregnant before
- Your uterus is an irregular shape
- Your babies are being delivered preterm

"What is a nonstress test, and how is it different for a woman carrying multiples?"

The nonstress test (NST) measures how babies' hearts respond to movement. (Just

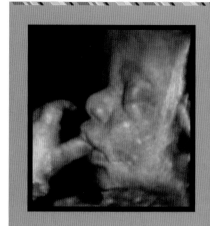

what babies are up to

- running out of room (no more somersaults)
- wedging feet in your ribs
- eyes dilate in response to light
- lungs are approaching maturity
- growth is starting to slow
- have creases on wrists and neck
- still plumping up
- brain still growing rapidly
- can recognize and react to music

like yours, your babies' heart rates should speed up when they wiggle.) While women carrying one child are rarely administered this test, moms-to-be of multiples are very likely to undergo an NST, since all multiple pregnancies are considered high risk. You'll take the test during the third trimester (as early as week 28), and depending on how many babies you're carrying and other clinical factors, you may go back into your doctor's office to do it a few more times before you deliver. If your OB schedules you for this test, take a potty break first—it can last up to an hour. You'll be hooked up to devices that will measure the babies' heart rates, and to monitors that will record the babies' movements. If any of your babies are sleeping, the OB may use a (totally safe!) buzzerlike instrument to wake 'em up. If one or more of your babies doesn't respond to movement with an accelerated heart rate, your OB may repeat the test or recommend

a biophysical profile to make sure the babies are okay in there.

❚ is it normal?

"My husband says I'm snoring now! Is this because I'm pregnant?"
Yes, pregnant women are more than twice as likely to snore as nonpregnant ones, and in the third trimester especially. Studies suggest that your new nighttime habit is due to more narrow upper airways, which should return to normal after delivery. There are also studies that link snoring in pregnancy to gestational diabetes, so it may be a good idea to let your OB know you're rattling the windows. And, as always, eat healthfully and exercise (heavier women are more likely to snore). If you didn't snore before pregnancy, you'll probably return to silent snoozing after the babies come.

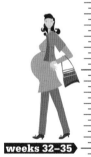

weeks 32–35

"I'm peeing a little every time I cough, sneeze, or laugh! What's going on?"

You bladder is shaped like a balloon with a little tube (your urethra) at the bottom to let out the urine. The muscles under your bladder usually keep that tube closed tight, but now there are bowling balls of babies pressing down on them, adding lots of pressure and putting those muscles to the test. And if they give way? Well, you leak pee. Don't worry, you've got a good defense: Kegels. In the meantime, a panty liner can at least help keep any leakage a secret.

delivery countdown

"What is my mucus plug? When can I expect it to come out?"

The mucus plug is the thick mucus your body uses to plug the opening of your cervix during pregnancy, sealing out bacteria and anything else harmful that could potentially make its way up to your babies. You might see it come out (it can look like a glob of snot and is sometimes tinged with blood) in the last month of pregnancy, or you might not see it at all. (For some women, it comes out in pieces or isn't very noticeable.) Your body will keep making mucus to fill its place, so you'll expel a good deal of discharge from now until delivery. If your mucus plug comes out more than three weeks before your due date, give your OB a call—she might want to check you out to make sure you aren't headed toward preterm labor. Don't get too excited if your

mucus plug comes out—while this definitely indicates your body's prep for labor, it doesn't really predict when labor will come. (Could be hours later. Could be weeks.)

"Will I be able to tell the difference between losing my mucus plug and my water breaking?"

Many a first-time mom has confused these two, especially since a ton of discharge can follow the loss of your mucus plug. Think of it this way: Mucus is gooey; water is liquid. So if it's thick, it's not your water. When your water breaks, it will be like . . . water. Amniotic fluid will trickle or gush and shouldn't have any color at all. It's possible, though, that the amniotic fluid will have a yellow, brown, or green tint—if so, be sure to let your OB know. This means one of the babies has pooped and will need to be monitored in case she's breathed it into her lungs.

"What is back labor? Will I have it?"

This is really just pain in your lower back as labor progresses. You'll usually feel it right above your tailbone. Sometimes, back labor seems to set in if one or more of your babies' heads is pressing against your tailbone, or if your babies are in awkward positions. But even if your little ones are perfectly packed in your womb, you may still experience back labor. A few (unlucky) women simply tend to feel labor in their back. Will you be one of them? There's no way to know until you go into labor. If you do feel the pain, try standing

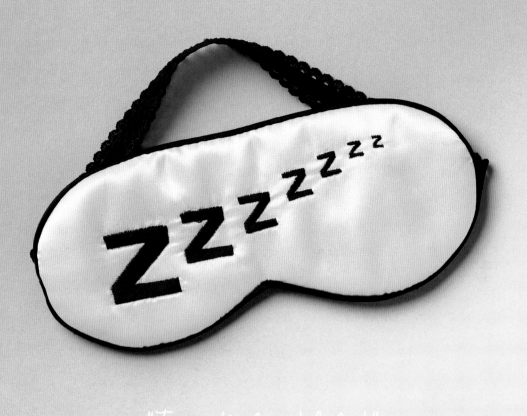

"I can't sleep! help!"

Between hormonal changes, a growing belly, a sore back, and a squished bladder, it's no wonder you're watching infomercials at 3 A.M. To help yourself catch some (much needed!) zzzs, use these tips to wind down and get comfy.

- Reduce your fluid intake after 7 P.M. (to cut down on bathroom runs).
- Read a book (not about pregnancy) to get your mind off your anxieties.
- Drink a small cup of chamomile tea before bed (known for its relaxing benefits).
- Stay active. Low-impact exercise can improve sleep.
- Ask your partner for a massage.
- Experiment with wedging pillows around your body to ease hip, back, or other pains.
- Take a warm bath.

weeks 32–35

under a warm shower, using hot or cold packs, shifting your position, having your mate massage you, or applying pressure with hands or a tennis ball. Of course, an epidural should do the trick too.

the day-to-day

"How do I decide between cloth and disposable diapers?"

The difference isn't as enormous as it used to be. Here's how they stack up:

HEALTH AND COMFORT No huge disparity, as long as you change your babies' diapers when they're full (a little more often with cloth). Leaving on a soiled diaper increases risk of diaper rash and isn't too pleasant for babies. Your babies might prefer the softer feel of cloth diapers. Disposable diapers are more breathable, but they can be stiff.

CONVENIENCE Forget the complicated folds and scary pins your mom had to deal with. Some cloth diapers come with Velcro or snap closures, fitted shapes, removable linings, and waterproof bands around the waist and legs, making the cloth change almost as quick and easy as the disposable. But cloth diapers aren't as absorbent, so you'll have to change them more often and do more laundry, or arrange for a diaper service.

PRICE Wash cloth diapers yourself and you'll save around $1,000 or more on your first child alone. The savings also depend on what sort of cloth diapers you purchase. (Prefolds are the least expensive option by far, while the sized, fitted—and cute!—versions can cost a pretty penny.) If you purchase secondhand diapers and/or save them for future children, your savings multiply. However, cloth diaper laundering services will set you back about the same amount as disposables—roughly $2,000 to $2,500 over three years.

ENVIRONMENT Not as clear cut as you might think. Yes, disposables use resources like trees and plastics during manufacturing, and then collect in landfills (most are 40 percent biodegradable). But consider the process of washing cloth diapers— clean water and energy are used, and nothing but dirty water is produced. (In other words, it's actually kind of a toss-up.) Note: For day care or travel, disposables win hands down. Studies show they reduce infection risk in a group setting—in fact, many day cares don't allow cloth. Cloth is too inconvenient on the road.

"Do I need to wash all of my babies' clothes before delivery?"

You should wash clothes (plus any blankets, sheets, and other fabrics) in dye- and scent-free detergent (skip the fabric softener and dryer sheets) before babies come home. Only wash a few of their clothes, and leave tags on the rest 'til you're positive that they'll be worn since there's no way to know your babies' sizes before delivery. (You can continue this tactic as your babies grow— they may not fit into those cute 6-month duds when they're 6 months old.)

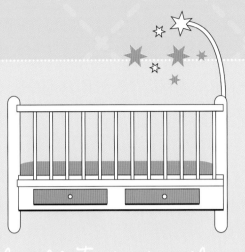

"should I start with a bassinet, rather than a crib?"

We know—you had one when you were little, your mother had one, your mother's mother had one . . . but unless you're getting a hand-me-down, it's probably not worth it, since you'll likely get only a few weeks' worth of use out of it before it starts to collect dust in the corner of the room. But if you do want one, get one—not two. Otherwise, try a travel crib or even a play yard (many come with a bassinet option)—you'll get more use out of them later on. Spend your time now looking for a good, solid crib.

Even if you choose to start out with a bassinet or a bedside sleeper, every baby needs a crib eventually. A few rules:

- Follow the assembly directions.
- It should be 100 percent sturdy, with no leftover pieces.
- Make sure slats are no more than 2⅜ inches apart so your babies can't get stuck.
- The mattress should fit securely against the sides.
- Look for a lowering feature so the mattress can be moved down as your babies grow.
- Only a waterproof pad and soft, fitted sheet are needed.
- Bumpers are a safety hazard (babies might get stuck under them and could suffocate).

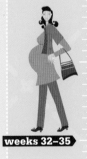

weeks 32–35

"how do I baby-proof my home?"

Your babies won't be mobile for several months, but there are some things you can do to keep them safe in the meantime . . . and to prepare for the day when they do get moving!

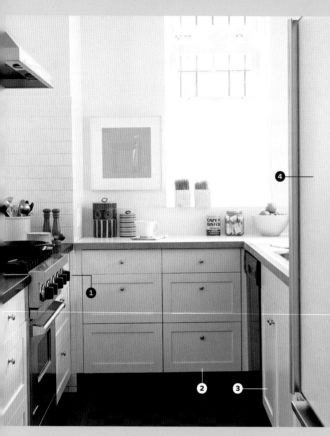
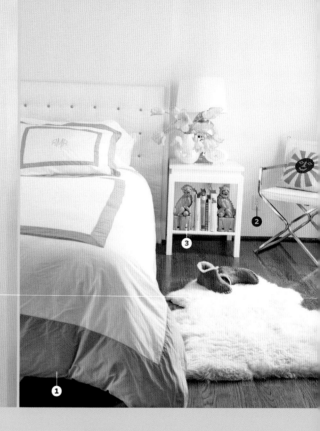

kitchen

1. Install stove guards and knob covers on oven.
2. Secure cabinets and drawers with latches.
3. Invest in a fire extinguisher; store in a cabinet near stove.
4. Move magnets off the fridge.

DON'T FORGET Use the back burners as much as possible and stow all cleaning items in high spots.

bedroom

1. Don't ditch your favorite duvet; cover with a sheet when babies are around.
2. Cover sockets with protectors.
3. Clear any exposed fragile items from nightstands.

DON'T FORGET Tame loose wires with cord clips and install window stops so windows open only 4 inches.

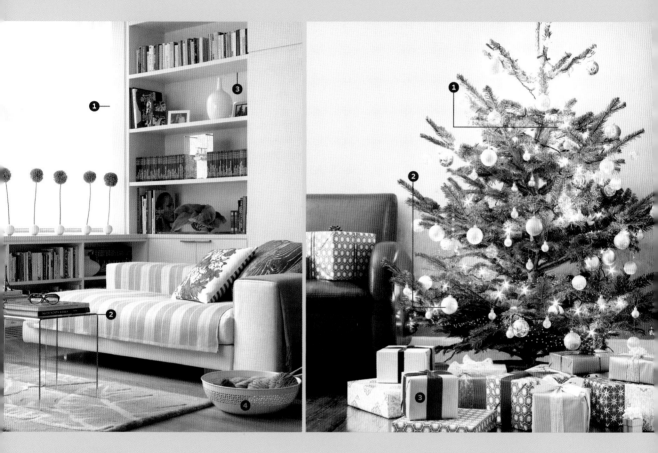

living room

1. Attach cord shorteners or wind-ups to window coverings.
2. Cushion sharp edges with guards.
3. Put brackets up high and out of reach.
4. Keep dangerous items off the floor.

DON'T FORGET Get a TV stand with a lip to prevent it from tumbling over. Put a secure gate in front of a fireplace.

holiday

1. Choose lead-free lights.
2. Hang fragile ornaments on higher branches.
3. Keep wrapped gifts off the floor. Ribbons and bows are choking hazards.

DON'T FORGET At the holidays, skip holly, amaryllis, mistletoe, and tinsel; they're harmful if eaten.

chapter

this is it—the final **1** *month and delivery!*

seven

almost there now By week 37 or 38, you should be about as big as you're going to get (hallelujah), and by week 38, you'll likely deliver (unlike your singleton-carrying friends, who typically go to week 39 or 40). Thirty-seven weeks marks a "full term" pregnancy, meaning babies are expected to thrive any time after that! These last weeks can really drag on, but try not to lose it—no baby stays in forever. Just think, after all this fuss about pregnancy, now the real adventure begins. Soon you'll help your babies find their way out of that giant belly and into your arms! Exciting, right? Here's the lowdown on what you're in for.

your to-do list

- Memorize the signs of labor
- Go on a date with your partner
- Make final preparations for babies
- Install the car seats
- Head to the hospital

Get more labor prep at TheBump.com/delivery

what you're in for...

"

I'm freaking out.

There's suddenly more room between my belly and my boobs.

I was terrified I'd poop during labor... and when the time came, I SO didn't care.

TONS OF DISCHARGE.

I think this is it!

Come on, babies...

My belly itches like crazy.

I WANT TO CLEAN ALL THE WINDOWSILLS WITH A Q-TIP. TWICE.

WHERE DID THIS SUDDEN SURGE OF ENERGY COME FROM?

hurry up!

Now I really can't sleep.

PLEASE LET THESE BABIES HAVE TINY HEADS.

OMG— MY WATER BURST!

"

on your mind...

❧ at the ob's office

"How do I decipher what the OB tells me about my progress in an exam?"

Your doctor will use four measures to help evaluate your progress:

RIPENING is the softening of your cervix. The cervix must ripen before it can thin or open.

EFFACEMENT is the thinning of the cervix. This is measured in percentage, with 0 percent meaning no thinning has occurred yet and 100 percent being as thin as you'll get.

DILATION is the opening of your cervix. This is measured in centimeters, from 0 to 10. (Ten is when the cervix has stretched to the diameter of the largest part of the babies' heads.)

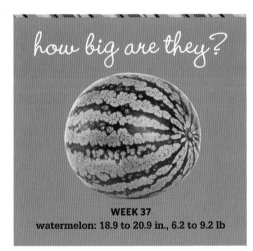

how big are they?

WEEK 37
watermelon: 18.9 to 20.9 in., 6.2 to 9.2 lb

STATION is the position of the babies' heads as it relates to the ischial spines (bony spots on each side of the pelvis). It's measured on a scale of -5 (head floating above the pelvis) to +5 (head crowning at the vagina's opening).

"Will I be able to tell my kids apart when they're down there?"

It depends on how far along you are and whether you're carrying more than two. Starting at about the 24-week mark, those babies can clearly establish their own territories. Often, baby A (so named because she's closest to the cervix and therefore likely to be born first) will stay on one side while baby B stays on the other. The less room they have, the less likely they are to move around. But baby A may switch with B without your even realizing it (see, they're playing games already!). By the way, while you may not always know which baby is which, your doctor, who is monitoring each one's progress, should be able to distinguish who's who and how well each one is doing.

"What's a contraction stress test?"

A contraction stress test is sometimes used to evaluate whether babies are in a strong enough condition to handle the stresses of labor. Most contraction stress tests are ordered to monitor the health of overdue babies. If yours are overdue, keep in mind that there is a fairly high rate of false positives (around 30 percent). How does the test work? Basically, two different devices strapped around your belly will separately record fetal heart rate and contractions, while an IV drip of oxytocin causes your uterus to contract. (Sometimes there's no IV, and you'll be taught how to stimulate your nipples to naturally coax the contractions instead.) If your babies are doing fine,

weeks 36+

their heart rates will be constant, or will briefly dip during contractions and return to normal quickly. However, if their heart rates slow with contractions and stay that way, it might indicate fetal distress (usually due to a problem with the placenta), and your doctor may recommend an immediate c-section or induction of labor.

"What is a biophysical profile, and how is it different for a woman carrying multiples? How often will this be administered?"

A biophysical profile is often administered to moms of multiples in the third trimester. The test combines an NST with an ultrasound examination that assesses the babies' body movements, muscle tone, breathing movements, and levels of amniotic fluid. Each baby will be tested individually and given points; a score between 8 and 10 is normal. If all looks good, your OB will likely repeat the test once or twice a week until delivery. If not, she may schedule you for more tests or suggest delivering the babies right away via induction or c-section.

"My doctor says I need to schedule a c-section. How and when do I do this?"

If your doctor has decided in advance that you'll need to deliver via c-section, his office will probably schedule the procedure for you as early as a few months in advance. The surgery should take place as close to your due date as possible—typically about two to three weeks prior for twins—since

you still want to prevent health problems that can be a result of preterm birth (like underdeveloped lungs). Even if your doc is taking care of the scheduling, you'll probably have to be in touch with the hospital yourself to fill out any preregistration paperwork required. You also should consider getting a tour of the hospital prior to the surgery, so you get to know the facilities.

"When will my OB start checking my cervix? Will she do it every time?"

Your OB will perform a pelvic examination during your first visit, but after that, the frequency of this exam varies, depending on the doctor, your health, and how many babies you're carrying. Your cervix's dilation and effacement might be checked every week starting at week 20 (or earlier!), or not until week 24, and then again within your third trimester. Ideally, your cervix will stay closed throughout the pregnancy until labor, but if you experience preterm labor or Braxton Hicks contractions, either of these may make the cervix shorten and the cervical walls thin, so your doctor will want to keep a close eye on you. If your cervix shortens or opens too early, your doctor may recommend a cervical cerclage, a procedure that sews the cervix closed to help prevent early delivery. If you're just curious about the status of your cervix and really want an internal exam, you can always request one from your OB.

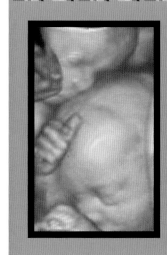

what babies are up to

- filling up your whole abdomen
- still adding padding
- brains still growing rapidly
- refining blinking and sucking skills
- practicing "breathing" amniotic fluid
- bowels are filling with meconium (babies' first poop)
- lungs are becoming fully mature
- flipping head-down to get ready to exit
- all systems are go

"What is 'stripping your membranes'? Does it really get labor going?"

To "strip" your membranes, your doctor will sweep her (gloved) finger over the thin membranes that connect the amniotic sac and your uterus. This prompts your body to release prostaglandins, hormones that ripen the cervix and can bring on contractions. This procedure won't be done unless you go past your due date, and even then it isn't guaranteed to work.

"Will my contractions be different because I'm carrying twins?"

About midway through your pregnancy, you may start to experience some Braxton Hicks contractions, or a tightening of the muscles of the uterus. They're generally not painful, just a little uncomfortable, and they last about a minute or two. When you're carrying twins or more, you'll typically have a greater number of Braxton Hicks, although some women don't have any symptoms. It's just your body's way of helping you get ready for the real thing. Actual labor contractions are similar for twins and singles (and yes, we're sorry to say, they hurt).

"What is premature rupture of membranes?"

The amniotic sac, also called the water bag, protects your babies from germs, bumps, and other hazards. If your water breaks early (before 37 weeks), that protective pod goes away, increasing the risk of infection and possibly causing early labor. When your uterus is carrying more than one passenger, your risk of preterm premature rupture of membranes (known as preterm PROM in medical circles) increases. You'll know it's

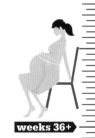

weeks 36+

happened if you wake up feeling wet or have lots of fluid in your bed, as if you've had an accident, or if you feel a sudden gush of fluid that keeps leaking. Call your doctor immediately if you experience any of these symptoms, or if you develop contractions, vaginal bleeding, or a fever.

Your doctor may treat this differently depending on how early the rupture occurs. If it's before 34 weeks, you may be placed on bed rest or hospitalized to decrease the amount of fluid loss. You may also be given antibiotics, steroids, or other medications to slow delivery and prevent complications. After 34 weeks, you're more likely to be sent to the delivery room, where you'll soon meet your newest family members.

in your head

"What if my OB isn't around on the day I go into labor?"

If you haven't asked your doctor who will deliver your babies in case she's not available, ask now. If you already have a good idea of who will be on call when your OB isn't and are simply panicking, settle down. Trust that your OB will leave you in good hands. Plus, you'll likely be spending more time with the labor nurses than with your OB.

"What if I think I'm in labor and the hospital sends me home?"

Well, you'll probably just get back in your car and go home. You might feel embarrassed, but the labor and delivery (or emergency room) staff are used to false alarms. Don't ignore labor symptoms for fear of being wrong; better to show up early than late!

"I am SO ready for these kids to come out. Can I safely induce labor at home?"

Here's an answer you won't like: not really. There are a few rumored remedies that you're welcome to try (taking a walk, eating spicy food, dancing, having sex), but don't get your hopes up that these will actually work. Other tactics (think: taking herbal supplements or castor oil, and stimulating your nipples) can do the trick, but we don't recommend them—they might bring on killer contractions that can be dangerous to your baby and super-painful to you. (Don't try these or any other methods without your midwife's or doctor's advice.)

"What if my due date goes right on by with no babies? Is missing your due date dangerous when carrying multiples?"

Your pregnancy time line is different from the projected schedule of your fellow moms-to-be who are carrying singletons. If you're pregnant with identical twins, your optimal delivery time is at 37 weeks, and if you're expecting fraternal twins, you should deliver by 38 weeks. Ideally, triplets should be born between 34 and 36 weeks and quadruplets between 30 and 32 weeks, depending on their size and lung capabilities. When you're pregnant with multiples, there is an increased chance of fetal loss or distress inside the womb after 39 weeks, so your doctor will likely recommend an induction if you still haven't gone into labor by then. The end is in sight!

is it normal?

"Why did I just feel like a lightning bolt shot through my vagina?"

This phenomenon doesn't seem very well documented, but we know many a mama who has complained of what we like to call "lightning crotch." What is it? Well, some women experience an occasional sharp pain in the pelvis or inside the vagina in the last weeks of pregnancy. This is probably related to your cervix dilating or to the pressure of the babies' heads on your cervix. (Either way, know that you're not alone.)

"I've heard moms talk about pooping during delivery. Is this common?"

Not everyone experiences this, but it's not at all unexpected. It's not usually very much, and the nurse just wipes it away. Trust us, it sounds like it would be humiliating, but you won't even care (or even necessarily know) when you're in the moment.

GREAT DEBATE

inducing labor: safe to stimulate?

natural labor is best

"When induction isn't necessary, it won't improve the labor outcome and can actually have the opposite effect. In our hospital, for women having their first baby, the c-section rate is 8 percent. If they're induced, it's 44 percent. If the woman's cervix isn't favorable and the baby isn't in a good position but you induce because of the calendar, you're inviting a c-section because you'll have a failed vaginal delivery." *Dr. Michael C. Klein, MD, CCFP, FAAP (Neonatal-Perinatal), FCFP, ABFP*

induction has benefits

"What I do is 'active management.' This means doing something about the risks rather than just simply waiting for something to happen. There aren't many situations where inducing can increase complications, as long as you're aware of the cervical status. Plus, there's the added benefit of a scheduled delivery. If women can have elective c-sections, then why not elective inductions?" *Dr. James M. Nicholson, MD*

Get more induction info at **TheBump.com/induction**

weeks 36+

▌is it safe?

"I'm full term anyway. Can I just ask the doctor to induce me already?"

Patience, child. Just because you are "full term" doesn't mean your babies are ready to come out. Your body knows when the time is right, and it's safer not to cut it short, especially before you've passed your due date. Plus, induction isn't without risks. Inducing labor too early (for example, if your due date projections were off) could result in a preterm birth, putting your babies at risk for health issues. Induction also increases the risk of infection (for you and your babies), umbilical cord problems, low fetal heart rates, the need for a c-section, and an increased risk of uterine rupture if you're trying for a VBAC (vaginal birth after cesarean).

"Is it still okay for me to take a bath after my water has broken?"

There are different opinions on this one (some experts worry about risk of infection), so ask your OB or midwife to be sure. Once your water breaks, you shouldn't really do anything without running it by your doctor first. In fact, she'll probably want you to call as soon as the amniotic sac springs a leak, and will probably ask you to come on in to the hospital, at least in the next few hours.

▌delivery countdown

"How can I tell if labor is coming soon?"

There's no real way to predict the moment when your body will post your babies'

eviction notice, and when you're expecting multiples, labor typically comes early, so it may be difficult to recognize the symptoms. Additionally, a mom-to-be often won't trust her own instinct that the big moment has arrived, so she will fail to act on her intuition. In this case, it's much better to be safe than sorry, so if you notice any indication of labor or suspect that the time has come, call your OB immediately. In the meantime, pay close attention to your body and watch for these signs:

NESTING Many women feel an overwhelming desire to clean and organize. The urges can be extreme (think scrubbing the bathroom grout with a toothbrush or rearranging the clothes in your closet).

LIGHTENING This is when the baby "drops," settling down into your pelvis. You may or may not notice that your bump has changed shape, your lungs have more room (you can breathe again), and you feel the pressure of your babies' heads in your pelvis (between your legs) . . . and on your bladder. As a mom-to-be of multiples, you have less room in that womb, so you may have been feeling this pressure for a few months already, but if it's a new sensation, that's a sign!

DIARRHEA Many women experience diarrhea within a few days of labor, thought by some to be the body's way of emptying out before it needs to do all that pushing.

STRONGER BRAXTON HICKS CONTRACTIONS Your "practice" contractions will probably get more uncomfortable within a couple of weeks of labor. (Remember: Real labor

"how should my babies be positioned for labor?"

If you're expecting triplets or more, it's almost certain that your babies will be delivered via c-section, so their positioning for labor is a nonissue. (It's very difficult to monitor the babies in the womb while one baby is being delivered, so most OBs will eliminate vaginal delivery as an option.)

But if you're birthing twins, there may be a chance you can deliver vaginally. If this is the case, baby A (the one that's coming out first) should be in a vertex position, which means head down and facing your side in the womb, but will come out facing your back. Her head will duck as she descends through the birth canal, so she'll come out crown first (hence the conehead look many newborns sport).

Once baby A is delivered, baby B is sometimes able to shift into a vertex position, but if baby B is transverse (on its side) or breech (feet or butt down), you may have to undergo a cesarean to get her out. In some cases, your OB will be able to turn baby B into a vertex position or, in other cases, will manage to deliver the baby breech.

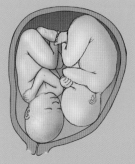
Vertex

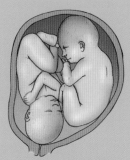
Vertex Breech

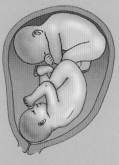
Transverse Breech

weeks 36+

contractions will get consistently stronger, longer, and more frequent.)

LOSING YOUR MUCUS PLUG The mucus plug often comes loose just before true labor sets in. It means progress—your body is making way for the babies.

A TON OF DISCHARGE After the mucus plug is expelled, you'll see a whole lot of clearish or whitish discharge.

BLOODY SHOW This pink-tinged discharge (as in blood from burst capillaries, plus the aforementioned discharge) means your cervix has started to thin and/or dilate. Labor should be on its way! (Call your OB immediately if you see bright-red blood that looks like a period.)

YOUR WATER BREAKS There's a chance that one or more of the membranous sacs that have been housing your babies will rupture and you'll feel fluid being released from your vagina. (It's not always a big burst; sometimes you'll just feel a trickle of water.) This doesn't happen for everyone; in fact, many moms deliver while these membranes are still intact. However, if your water does break, call your OB immediately; even if you don't go into labor, you will likely be induced to prevent fetal infection.

"If I bleed during my last few weeks of pregnancy, am I going into labor?"

Maybe, but not always. If you're seeing blood-tinged mucus (aka "bloody show") along with other signs of labor, like contractions, pressure in your pelvis or lower abdomen, or a dull lower backache, your babies may be gearing up for arrival. Light bleeding in late pregnancy could also be a sign of common conditions like cervical growths or inflammation. Call your OB right away if you see any bright-red blood or experience heavy bleeding— this could signal a problem.

"What is a version?"

A cephalic version is a technique an OB uses to attempt to shift babies into the proper birthing position. Basically, your doc will push and prod your breech or transverse baby to try and get him vertex. For singletons, this may happen in the weeks before labor (but almost never before week 36), but for moms of twins, it's often done during labor to prepare the babies to be delivered vaginally. First, your doctor will perform an ultrasound to determine baby's position and heart rate, the placenta's position, and the amount of amniotic fluid. In an external version, the doctor (and maybe a helper) will push or lift your tummy to try and help baby roll into position. In an internal version, the OB will enter through the vagina with her hands in an attempt to turn the baby. She may use an ultrasound to guide her in the procedure, and to keep track of your babies' heart rates. And yes, even if your OB does manage to get baby into position, he could still flip back. The good news: More than half of version attempts are successful, so it's worth a shot, and complications from this procedure are rare.

"Anything I can do to get my babies to turn?"

Unfortunately, there's no surefire way to make your babies shift. If there were, we would rarely see breech babies. Still, there are a couple of things you can try. (These aren't proven effective, but they aren't total hogwash, either—both methods seemed to turn a number of fetuses in scientific studies.)

KNEE-CHEST POSITION Before you attempt this, ask your doctor if it's safe for you; make sure you describe this method completely and accurately to your OB and get the green light before trying it: Get on your hands and knees (in a crawling position) on the bed, and lay your head, shoulders, and chest flat on the mattress. If your belly is pressed against your thighs, scoot your knees back until it's hanging free. Hold for 15 minutes, and repeat every two hours while awake.

MOXIBUSTION Some acupuncturists believe that burning an herb called moxa (aka mugwort) near your little toe may urge fetuses to flip. (Nope, we're not kidding.)

"What do contractions feel like? How much do they hurt?"

Since contractions are experienced slightly differently by different women, we can't really tell you. (Afraid we were going to say that, weren't you?) Some women describe contractions as feeling like super-intense menstrual cramps;

others of us feel a dull ache in our backs that wraps around to the front; and still others only feel a sharp pain in our backs, or only an intense pain in our bellies. Early contractions can also feel like a terribly upset stomach (diarrhea and all), or you might feel contractions radiating through your thighs. When asked to rate the degree of the pain, mamas-to-be also give drastically different answers, though the pain should always increase in intensity as labor progresses. And while chances are slim that this will be a near-painless experience (childbirth hurts—you knew that), you may be surprised to find the pain far easier—or, yes, far tougher—to deal with than you're imagining. This pain has a purpose—you hurt because your uterine muscles are working hard to push your babies into the world.

"How do I time contractions? Are there any tools to help?"

To time contractions, you'll pay attention to and record two things:
- The time each contraction begins
- How long each contraction lasts

This will tell you the frequency and duration of your contractions. (Note: To find out how "far apart" your contractions are, measure from the beginning of one contraction to the beginning of the next—NOT the time between them.) Your OB will probably give you a guideline for when to call or head to the hospital (like, when contractions are 5 minutes

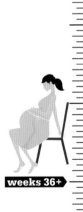

weeks 36+

apart and lasting 30 to 45 seconds). Keep track the old-fashioned way with a stopwatch and a piece of paper (if you're really in labor, you'll probably need your mate to help). Or use an online contraction counter (we have one at TheBump.com/tools), and there are even a few iPhone applications that can help. Either way, you'll be looking for contractions that last progressively longer and come closer together. Each contraction might not be longer, or arrive sooner, than the one before it, but in true labor, a pattern will form over the course of a few hours.

"How do I know if I'm in labor for real or if it's false labor?"

When actual labor sets in, contractions get longer, stronger, and closer together—and they won't stop or decrease in intensity if you walk around or change position. You'll also see a bloody show (heavy discharge that's pinkish or blood-streaked), and, of course, it's possible that your water will break.

With false labor, however, contractions won't be regular (you might have three that are 4 minutes apart, and then nothing for 20 minutes). They also won't get closer together or progressively more painful, and should ease up if you get up and walk, or change positions. You might also feel your babies moving around during the contractions (but call your OB if they seem frantic). If you see blood in false labor, it should be brownish (probably from an internal exam or from having had sex in the past day or two).

"When will my water break?"

Imagining that scene in every movie and television show, where the woman's water breaks at the same instant that contractions set in? Don't count on this happening to you. Only about 10 percent of women have their membrane rupture before labor begins. So you could be in that 10 percent, or your water could break sometime during labor, or your doctor might wind up breaking your water for you on the delivery table.

"I'm scheduled for a c-section and am nervous about the anesthesia. What are my options?"

For a c-section, the choices are an epidural block, a spinal block, or general anesthesia. You may or may not have a choice—your OB may take your preferences into account, but she'll ultimately make a decision based on both your and your babies' well being. If you're put under general anesthesia, you won't be awake for the cesarean. With the epidural and spinal blocks, the lower half of your body will be numbed for the surgery, but you'll remain awake. Try not to worry about it too much. Yes, all three anesthesia options will involve a needle, but the needle prick is guaranteed to be less painful than what you'd feel without it! Women have c-sections every day—and no matter how you're numbed, you'll be meeting your babies in no time.

chart

contraction counter

Think you're going into labor? Keep track of your contractions with our easy-to-use Contraction Counter. Or try the digital one at TheBump.com.

	start time	stop time	length of contraction	frequency of contraction
1	:	:		
2	:	:		
3	:	:		
4	:	:		
5	:	:		
6	:	:		
7	:	:		
8	:	:		
9	:	:		
10	:	:		
11	:	:		
12	:	:		
13	:	:		
14	:	:		
15	:	:		
16	:	:		
17	:	:		
18	:	:		
19	:	:		
20	:	:		

weeks 36+

"Are there differences between multiple-pregnancy labors and singleton labors?"

Every pregnancy and every labor is different, but just because you're having multiples doesn't mean you'll have double the pain. Phew! In some ways, you may even be getting off a little easier—multiple babies for the price of just one labor. As for the actual delivery, the likelihood of having a c-section greatly increases with each additional baby, but many twins are born vaginally. In this scenario, you're going to have to push twice, once for each baby, and there will likely be 15 to 20 minutes between the two births. So, after baby number one arrives, you'll have to muster some additional strength.

"Should I be worried about the cord wrapping around my baby's neck?"

It's certainly not uncommon. The umbilical cord winds up around a baby's neck in about 25 percent of deliveries, but usually it stays loose and causes no harm. Your OB will simply use a finger to slip the cord over baby's head at birth, or will clamp and cut it if it's wrapped too snugly. Sometimes, this can be a dangerous condition, particularly when the cord gets wrapped or knotted so tightly that it cuts off baby's blood supply. A decrease in fetal activity or an abnormal heart rate during labor may be signs of a troublesome nuchal cord. Nuchal cords occur only when babies are delivered vaginally, so if you are pregnant with triplets or more and you're likely getting a c-section, you don't

have to worry about this at all. One less concern for you!

"What is an episiotomy? Is it likely that I'll have to have one?"

An episiotomy is an incision made in the perineum (the skin between the vagina and the anus) during labor to help allow the baby to be delivered with greater ease. This procedure used to be very common but is considered passé by many OBs today. In fact, the number of episiotomies administered within the United States has decreased substantially within the last decade. Sometimes an OB will perform an episiotomy to deliver a baby more quickly when there are signs of fetal distress. If your doctor decides you need an episiotomy, you'll receive a local anesthetic (unless your perineum is already numb from the pressure of the babies' heads or from an epidural). Then your OB will make a small slice in your perineum, and once your babies are delivered, you'll get another shot of anesthesia (you'll feel a pinch) and a few stitches, which should disintegrate in a matter of weeks.

"In what scenario might I have to have an emergency c-section?"

In general, emergency c-sections are called for if anything happens to put you or your babies in danger. As discussed before, if you're pregnant with triplets or more, your doctor will likely already have scheduled a c-section, but if you're expecting twins and plan on delivering vaginally, an emergency c-section may still be an option if your doctor feels it's best. In some cases, the first baby will be delivered vaginally and the second baby will be delivered via cesarean, or it's possible that you could undergo a c-section for both babies, even if your birth plan doesn't call for it. Any time fetal distress is present or your health is at risk, your doc may decide to perform surgery. Some potential risks that may lead to an emergency c-section are: prolapsed cord (in which the umbilical cord comes out ahead of the baby), placental abruption (when the placenta begins to come loose, causing you and the baby to lose blood), and/or breech or traverse positioning (in which the baby or babies are not positioned head down for delivery). You may also wind up with an emergency c-section if your labor stops progressing or takes way too long, particularly if your water has broken, which makes the babies more susceptible to infection.

"What is the likelihood that my multiples will need to stay in the NICU?"

Since multiples have a much higher rate of prematurity than singletons, there's a greater risk that your babies won't be fully developed at delivery, which means they'll need special care in the NICU before they can go home. How long they stay in the NICU will depend on a number of factors, including gestation at delivery, weight, any complications, and the overall health of the babies. But try not to be too overwhelmed by the NICU—it's just a place for your babies to receive extra-special care.

the big day

"What will happen when I get to the hospital or birthing center?"

The exact routine depends on your hospital's specific procedures, but odds are, it will go something like this: First, you'll check in (if you preregistered, this will take only a second). Next, you'll have the dilation of your cervix checked to make sure you're in active labor. Then you'll be taken to the OR or the birthing room (even if you plan to deliver vaginally, you may be taken to the OR, just in case your doc needs to perform a last-minute c-section, as often happens with multiples) and admitted—you'll be having babies today!

Once in the room, you'll be quizzed about your status (when your contractions started, how far apart they are, if your water has broken), given a lovely, butt-baring hospital gown, and asked to sign some routine consent forms. Once you hop (okay, maybe not hop, exactly) onto the bed, the nurse will check your vitals (pulse, blood pressure, temperature, breathing), may check your cervix, will look for anything leaking out (like blood or amniotic fluid), and will monitor your babies' heart rates with a Doppler or fetal monitor. Your babies will likely each be monitored consistently to ensure they are doing well. Your babies' positions will be

weeks 36+

real moms uncensored

on pain relief...

> I wanted to go natural, but I ended up being induced and the Pitocin was too much for me to take, so I got the epidural. *ahnella*

> It took them seven attempts and I had a monster bruise afterward, but it was worth it! *MrsErinnElizabeth*

> The epidural was a breeze going in. Didn't feel a thing getting it. I could still move my legs and was pretty mobile in bed. *dle927*

> I was afraid of the epidural, but once I had it, I was in heaven. Three hours of pushing, forceps, and an episiotomy—I didn't feel a thing! Heaven! *krissyh21*

checked too, and you may be hooked up to IV fluids at this point (this is routine in some hospitals but not in others).

"What are my pain relief options for a vaginal delivery?"

There are several ways to lessen discomfort during labor and delivery.

SYSTEMIC ANALGESICS These are drugs that are injected into your muscle or a vein and work on your whole nervous system to relieve (but not erase) your pain. They might make you tense or nauseated, so sometimes you'll receive another drug to relieve the side effects. Systemic analgesics are given more often early in labor—if they're given too close to delivery, babies can come out with slower reflexes and breathing.

EPIDURAL BLOCK An epidural block involves injecting analgesics (that numb you partially for a vaginal delivery) or anesthetics (that numb you more completely for a c-section, or if your OB needs to use forceps or a vacuum) into a space below your spinal cord known as the "epidural space." First they'll numb you up with an injection of local anesthesia, and then the epidural needle will be inserted. The anesthesiologist will probably thread a little tube through the needle and leave it in as a way to give you more epidural meds later in labor—or you might receive the drugs continuously. Your bottom half will be moderately numb within 10 to 20 minutes, and the degree of numbness can be adjusted. Epidural side effects include reduced blood pressure, shivering, and headaches. Rarely,

"can you help me understand the stages of labor?"

Sure. There's a lot that happens, and no two labors are the same, but here's the status quo:

stage 1

This stage is the longest and is divided into 3 phases of its own.

EARLY LABOR Your cervix effaces (thins) and dilates from 0 cm to 3 cm. Mild to moderate contractions set in, coming every 5 to 20 minutes and lasting 30 to 60 seconds.

TO DO
- Rest or nap
- Have a light snack
- Pee frequently (a full bladder slows labor)
- Double-check your hospital bag
- Time contractions

ACTIVE LABOR Your cervix opens from 3 cm to 7 cm. Your contractions get more intense, coming every 3 to 4 minutes and lasting 40 to 60 seconds each. You'll head to the hospital as this phase begins.

TO DO
- Practice your breathing exercises
- Try to relax between contractions
- Keep peeing at least once an hour
- Walk around if you can
- Get pain relief, if you want it

TRANSITION Your cervix dilates to 10 cm. Contractions will last 2 to 3 minutes and come every 60 to 90 seconds.

TO DO
- Use your breathing exercises
- Don't push until your OB says to
- Try to stay focused

stage 2

This stage begins when you're fully dilated. Contractions will probably stay around 60 to 90 seconds, but may be farther apart (usually 2 to 5 minutes). You'll want to push.

TO DO
- Breathe—your babies need your oxygen
- Try to stay (relatively) calm and focused
- Concentrate on relaxing any tense body parts
- Get into a position that uses gravity to your best advantage
- Go with the flow—your body knows what to do
- Rest between contractions
- Ask for a mirror if you want to see just what is happening down there
- Push with all your might!

stage 3

After the babies arrive, your uterus will contract again (mildly) to kick out the placenta. This lasts 5 to 10 minutes but can take up to 30. Once that's out, your OB will stitch up any tears or your episiotomy, and labor is done!

TO DO
- Push if the doctor asks you to
- Thank your coach for the support
- Relax and enjoy your babies

weeks 36+

the meds can enter a vein and cause a seizure or dizziness. They can also enter your spinal fluid and affect your chest muscles, making it hard to breathe (also rare).

SPINAL BLOCK A spinal block goes in through your lower back too, but with a much smaller needle, and your lower half is instantly numbed. It lasts only an hour or two, so you probably want to save it up for pushing time. Side effects are the same as with an epidural.

COMBINED SPINAL-EPIDURAL BLOCK Also known as a "walking epidural," the combined block is injected into both the spinal fluid and the space below the spinal cord. You'll have instant relief, and can have more drugs through the epidural for pain relief all the way through delivery. And yes, you might be able to walk around once the block is in place.

GENERAL ANESTHESIA General anesthesia knocks you out cold. You probably won't receive this unless you wind up needing an emergency c-section and a spinal block or epidural isn't possible or practical, for some reason. If you need to be put under, the meds will cause you to lose consciousness quickly, and the anesthesiologist will put a breathing tube down your windpipe after you're out.

ALTERNATIVE THERAPIES If you'd rather skip the meds, you may find relief through self-hypnosis, soaking in water, transcutaneous electrical nerve stimulation (or TENS—a therapy that uses little electrical jolts to reduce pain), meditation, or Lamaze.

"One of my babies is still breech—I'm definitely going to have a c-section, right?"
Most OBs will recommend a cesarean, but a vaginal birth might still be an option too, especially if a version (turning the baby manually) is successful. When your due date nears and baby is still breech, you and your OB will inevitably discuss both the risks and benefits of giving a version—or even a breech delivery—a shot.

"Will the doctor break my water?"
If your water (aka "amniotic sac," "bag of waters," or "membranes") hasn't broken on its own when you arrive at the hospital, and you're dilated 5 centimeters or more, your OB might recommend bursting the bag by hand—especially if your cervix seems to be making slow (or no) progress. (Some OBs will go ahead and break your water at 3 or 4 centimeters.) The reasoning behind this: "Artificial rupture of membranes" (popping a hole in the amniotic sac) will usually jump-start labor by getting serious contractions under way. If labor is moving along fine, you and your doctor might decide to wait this one out—after all, contractions tend to be more painful after your water breaks. If the OB doesn't rupture your membranes, the sac will probably break on its own during labor, though once in a while it stays intact until babies make an exit. (Either way is fine.)

To break your water, the doctor will reach up and prod it with something that

delivery room

headwalls Just behind the bed on the headwalls, you will find the nurse call system, oxygen, suction, and air for you and your babies.

hemodynamic monitor This monitor measures your heart rate, blood pressure, and O_2 saturation.

fetal monitor A strap will be placed around your belly with two monitors—one tracks the babies' heart rate; the other tracks your contractions.

radiant heat warmer This device helps to keep your babies' temperature regulated after birth and during the initial assessment.

bed The entire bottom drops out and the stirrups come up when it's time to deliver. The bed might also have handlebars to hold on to as you push.

patient care cart This holds all the supplies needed for labor, including peri-pads, IV supplies, gauze, and slippers.

partition To give you privacy during the actual birth and to block off what's going on outside your room if you need to rest during a long labor.

looks like a crochet hook. You might feel (very little) discomfort as the device enters your vagina, but as for the actual water breaking, most women feel only a big, warm gush of liquid.

"How will they make sure my babies are okay during labor?"

DOPPLER If your pregnancy is low risk and your babies have been doing A-OK so far, your OB or nurses might simply keep tabs on the babies' heart rates with a fetal Doppler monitor (the same way they listen to your babies at your prenatal appointments). If that's the case, they'll probably check in at least every half-hour before you start pushing, and then every 5 minutes during delivery.

EXTERNAL FETAL MONITOR Intermittent monitoring can be time-consuming, so you might have a fetal monitor strapped to your bump instead. (This is routine in many hospitals.) The monitor consists of two small devices, one that tracks your contractions, and one that tracks your babies' heartbeats. Both will be hooked to a monitor that will print out the data or display it on a screen (the same info may be on display for doctors or nurses down the hall). You may have these strapped around you during the whole labor.

INTERNAL FETAL MONITOR If your doctor feels the need to keep a closer watch on your babies' status (especially if she thinks your babies may be in distress), she may reach up and stick electrodes on their heads.

(Clearly, you'll have to be a little dilated first, and your water must be broken.) The electrode tracks the babies' heart rates, and you may also have a little tube (aka catheter) stuck into your uterus to gauge the contractions. Sometimes they skip the catheter and monitor contractions with the external device on your tummy. There are a few small risks involved, like irritation or infection, or sometimes even an abscess or, rarely, a bald spot where the electrode is placed, so you won't have an internal monitor unless there is a clear need for it.

"I don't remember anything from my hospital tour. What should I know?"

Hospitals vary in their delivery room setup— some will keep you in one room the entire time, while others have a room specifically for delivery and then will move you to a separate recovery room. Some hospitals have delivery rooms specially designed to be comfortable and soothing, while others feel more like . . . well, hospital rooms. It's a very good idea to take a tour before you go, so that you feel comfortable and you're prepared for whatever your situation is. Take notes.

"What medical staff will be in the room when I deliver?"

Good question—it's nice to be prepared for who'll be hanging around (and staring at your naughty bits) when you're in the delivery room. Hospitals have varied policies on what staff is present, but here's a rundown on the basics.

"what exactly are these tools and how are they used?"

Don't be alarmed when you see a nurse don a sterile hat, mask, and gloves. This means you're getting close to delivery and it's time to set up the doctor's table. Nothing's suddenly gone wrong—the nurse is simply keeping things sterile. Here's what's being set up:

forceps We admit, they look a little scary. These are generally used to try and shift babies' position, and may also help guide the head out.

vacuum If pushing is proving ineffective, your doc will use this to pull the babies out with suction. Don't be alarmed.

hemostat This clamp is used for containing any type of bleed, holding sutures, and—most important—cutting babies' umbilical cord.

amniotic hook It looks a lot scarier than it feels, we promise. This long crochet-like hook is used in the early stages of delivery to break your water if it hasn't yet happened naturally.

scalpel Unless you're having a c-section, your doctor probably won't use this—but it's kept on hand.

scissors Just in case you (Sorry! Really!) need an episiotomy.

you'll also see

SPONGE HOLDERS These rings are simply used to hold gauze.

LAPAROSCOPIC SPONGES If you start to bleed, your doc will hold these down to control it.

BUCKETS OF STERILE WATER Used to keep everything clean throughout the delivery.

SUTURES Your doc will use these to stitch you up if you tear or have an episiotomy.

weeks 36+

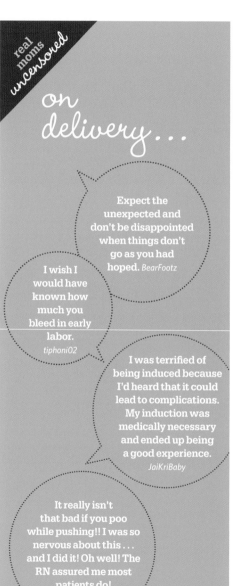

real moms uncensored

on delivery...

Expect the unexpected and don't be disappointed when things don't go as you had hoped. *BearFootz*

I wish I would have known how much you bleed in early labor. *tiphoni02*

I was terrified of being induced because I'd heard that it could lead to complications. My induction was medically necessary and ended up being a good experience. *JaiKriBaby*

It really isn't that bad if you poo while pushing!! I was so nervous about this . . . and I did it! Oh well! The RN assured me most patients do! *sprice88*

LABOR AND DELIVERY NURSE Your line of communication with your delivery practitioner and your support system. She's the one who monitors your progress and checks on the babies as you dilate. You might have the same nurse for your entire labor, or there could be one or more switches in staff due to shift changes.

DOCTOR OR MIDWIFE This is the person who delivers your babies. It may or may not be the one whom you've been seeing throughout your pregnancy (for example, your OB may be on vacation on the day you go into labor or be part of a practice that rotates which doctor is on call each day).

ANESTHESIOLOGIST If you'll receive pain relief during labor (spinal, epidural, or other meds), an anesthesiologist and/or nurse anesthetist may be present to drug you up.

OB TECH Sometimes an OB tech will come in just before delivery to assist the doctor or midwife and set up any instruments.

OTHER NURSE(S), SPECIALISTS, STUDENTS Depending on the hospital and the circumstances that surround your birth, there may be other staff present, like a nursery nurse, neonatologist, or medical student. You might also choose to have a doula present to offer emotional support.

"What are some good positions to try to make labor easier?"
Different positions feel different to different women, so experiment to find what feels right for you. That being said, here are some tried-and-true ones:

GET DOWN ON YOUR HANDS AND KNEES This position is good for relieving back labor.
HAVE YOUR PARTNER SIT IN A CHAIR WITH HIS LEGS APART Stand between his legs with your butt facing him, and go into a squat with your thighs spread apart (imagine making room for babies). Then, drape your arms over his knees to support yourself, and ask for a shoulder massage.
STAND FACING YOUR PARTNER, WITH YOUR ARMS AROUND HIS NECK Lean into him, or hang from his shoulders, and sway. This uses gravity to your advantage and gives you a break so that you don't have to hold all your own weight, and the movement helps get you through some seriously painful contractions.
LIE ON YOUR LEFT SIDE This is a great way to rest between contractions, and maximizes blood (and oxygen) flow to babies.

"Why do I need an IV during labor?"
For the most part, an IV is put in place so that there is a way to immediately plug any medicines into your bloodstream if it becomes necessary. Your OB might also use a drip of IV fluids to keep you hydrated during labor. (Just in case any medicines are ordered without your knowledge, always ask what is being sent through your IV line, or have your labor coach read the bag.)

"What does it mean if the doctor says I have a 'lip' left when she checks me?"
Basically, this term means that you're fully dilated, but an edge of your cervix (usually the anterior—or front—of the cervix) is a little bit swollen and is still in the way of your babies' heads. Your OB may wait until it moves into the correct position on its own, or she may try to pull it out of the way with her fingers while you bear down to push the babies past. Just be sure to wait until your doctor gives the okay to push—pushing against an anterior lip can make the swelling worse . . . and make it more difficult to get babies out.

"What is an Apgar score?"
The Apgar test is performed almost immediately after each of your babies is born to determine their health. Each baby will be tested individually 1 minute after birth and again 5 minutes after birth. The medical staff will evaluate activity, muscle tone, pulse, grimace response (reaction to stimulation—like a pinch), appearance (complexion), and respiration. Each of these will get a score from 0 to 2 (with 2 being the best score), and then those scores will be added up to a total. The point of the Apgar is to check whether any of your babies needs immediate medical care. Generally, a score over 7 is considered healthy. A lower score may mean that baby needs special attention—or she may just need a little time. No need to mention your babies' Apgars on their birth announcements; the test is a tool for your doctors and isn't meant to have anything to do with your babies' future health, intelligence, or behavior. Your doctor will let you know if there is any cause for concern.

weeks 36+

"What is a prolapsed cord?"

A prolapsed cord is when the umbilical cord manages to get in the way of a baby's exit and slips into the birth canal first—usually when the water breaks. Baby can push against the cord during labor, compressing it so that less oxygen is making its way to your little one. This is very dangerous for a baby, and might require an emergency c-section. If you think you can feel the cord in your vagina after your water breaks, get on your hands and knees (to reduce as much pressure on the cord as possible) in the back seat of the car while someone rushes you to the hospital, or call 911. Your doctor will most definitely want to get your babies out right away.

Prolapsed cords are more likely to occur with premature labors or with breech vaginal deliveries, but they are very rare (about 1 in 1,000 deliveries), so your chances of having to deal with this are slim.

"What will the placenta and umbilical cord look like when I deliver them?"

The umbilical cord looks like a flexible, spongy, twisted tube, consisting of two arteries and a vein covered in a whitish, see-through jelly. The placenta can be described as "cake-like," and is also spongy. It's big, bloody, veiny, and lumpy, with one red side (the side that was attached to your uterus) and one gray or silver side (the side that faced your babies for all those months).

"What happens during a c-section?"

Whether your cesarean is scheduled ahead due to complications or your babies' position (or, yes, even personal preference) or you're wheeled into the OR for an emergency c-section, the basics are the same:

First, a nurse will prep you for the surgery. This entails washing (and maybe shaving) your abdomen, and you might be given medication to reduce stomach acid so that it doesn't enter your lungs. You'll also receive an IV in your arm or hand, to pump you with any meds and fluids during the procedure. A catheter (a thin plastic tube) will be put in your bladder to empty it during surgery, which lowers your risk of injury, and you'll receive anesthesia (either an epidural, a spinal, or general anesthesia—see pages 132 and 134). Oh, and you get to wear a hairnet. (Are you brimming with excitement yet?)

In most cases, your partner will be able to join you for the surgery—he'll just have to wash up and don a snazzy set of sterile scrubs beforehand, along with a mask and hairnet. And don't worry about getting squeamish—you'll probably have a little curtain across your chest, blocking your view of all the exciting action.

Once you're under (or numbed), the OB will make either a vertical or transverse (aka horizontal) incision above your pubic hairline, going through your skin and abdomen. (The muscles can be moved, so, in most cases, they don't need to be cut.) Then another incision—again either vertical or transverse—is made in your uterine wall. Because they're done on the lower, thinner part of the uterus and thus you'll bleed less and heal better, transverse incisions are usually the first option. However, in some specific circumstances, such as a very preterm baby not yet in the head-down position, a vertical incision may be necessary.

Next comes the fun part: The doctor will gently pull your babies out through these incisions! Just after delivery, the doctor (or your partner) will cut the umbilical cord, and the placenta will be removed. Your uterus will be closed with dissolvable stitches, and more stitches or staples will close up your skin. You may or may not get to hold your babies for a few seconds—depending on their perceived health (and whether you're conscious)—but, barring any major health issues, you'll soon meet again the recovery room, where you can begin oohing and aahing over your bundles of joy.

"What will my babies look like when they finally come out?"

Sure, all newborns are beautiful miracles. But as far as aesthetics go, well, they tend to look like little larvae that just squeezed through a tight, slimy tube after soaking in fluid for 9 months. If your babies are born vaginally, they might have coneheads (c-section babies don't usually suffer this fate). And no matter the exit route, babies are likely to be wrinkly and might have swollen genitals and breasts, a coating of cheese-like vernix caseosa, a little fur (languno) on their backs and heads, poofy eyes, scratches, rashes, and other blotches and skin weirdness. But don't worry—they'll be gorgeous in their own way, and will come to look much more like chubby Gerber babies in a couple of months' time.

"What will happen to my babies in the hours after delivery?"

The routine differs depending on the hospital and doctor, but it usually goes something like this: Once your babies are out, your OB will clamp and cut (or let your partner cut) the cords. (Your babies will probably be lying on your tummy or chest for this.) Next, the OB will check their APGAR scores, give your babies a good rubdown with a towel, weigh and measure them, and give you and your babies matching wrist and/or ankle bands. Your babies will also get eye ointment to prevent infection, and will probably be wrapped up really tight to keep warm. You'll probably get to cuddle with your new additions for a while, and you may be able to give breastfeeding a go. (Your babies may or may not be ready to eat right away, though.)

After you've smothered your wee ones in kisses (and taken a million pictures), they'll probably head to the newborn nursery for their first bath, their first pediatrician visit (for a thorough checkup), footprints (if they weren't taken in the delivery room), a routine heel stick (for government-required blood work), a hepatitis B shot, and possibly other

weeks 36+

protective procedures. Your partner may be able to join your babies for the whole deal—just ask. If all is well, your babies will be deposited back in your arms once they're fully evaluated and swaddled up nice and tight.

"How long will I have to stay in the hospital?"

If you have a totally smooth vaginal birth, you're likely to head home within 24 to 48 hours after delivery. However, if you had a cesarean or any complications during delivery, you'll have to stick around for a while. (A typical c-section stay is about three days.) Use your time in the hospital to get some sleep and make sure you take advantage of the available support, like lactation and baby-care classes.

In some cases, your babies may have to stay longer than you, particularly if they are premature or need NICU care.

"Can moms of multiples always breast-feed right away?

You know how in the movies or on TV, no sooner is the cord cut than the newborn baby is immediately brought to nuzzle on mom's breast? There's a really good chance that's not going to happen to you. And that's OK: It's just that because the vast majority of twins (and almost all triplets) don't go the

---

GREAT DEBATE

circumcision... should you snip?

foreskin should stay

"Circumcision is unnecessary, risky, traumatic, and harmful. Also, all of the 'health' reasons for getting one have been debunked. It's painful, and the emotional trauma is stored deep in the brain. Severe bleeding can occur, and every year babies actually die from the procedure. Plus, there are chronic complications that might appear later, erectile dysfunction for one. Many people feel that it violates human rights." *Dr. Mark D. Reiss, MD*

snip the skin

"Circumcision is a very valuable preventative measure. A male who's uncircumcised has 10 times the risk of contracting a urinary tract infection during the first year of his life (when they're most dangerous). He's 3 times as likely to get HPV, which causes penile and cervical cancer. In fact, nearly 100 percent of penile cancer cases are in uncircumcised men." *Dr. Edgar Schoen, MD*

▶ Weigh in on snipping at **TheBump.com/circumcision**

full 40-week term, they're often swept away to the neonatal intensive care unit (NICU) to make sure breathing, heart rate, and all the other vitals are going A-OK. So that just means you may have to do your bonding a little later, in a slightly different atmosphere, surrounded by lots of little ones who need a little extra help. Don't worry if your new bunch isn't able to breastfeed immediately—often you may find the suck reflex isn't quite so fully developed, which can make it difficult for baby to latch onto breast. If you want to breastfeed (and all signs point to it being a very, very good thing for you and your babies), it's important to start pumping milk as soon as possible to get your milk supply going. Beyond feeding, most NICUs will encourage "kangaroo care" for premature infants: It's a chance to snuggle up close with your baby, giving him as much skin to skin contact as possible. (Bonus: Your partner can do this, too, no breasts required). Research shows this one-on-one contact can help stabilize your baby's heart and breathing rates, improve the amount of oxygen he's getting, and help regulate his body temperature. Babies who get kangaroo care also seem to get more sleep time, gain weight more rapidly, cry less, breastfeed more easily, and—best of all—come home earlier.

"I really want to breastfeed. Is there anything special I need at home?"

In theory, you'd think two breasts would really be all you'd need to get the job done. But in reality, all moms—and especially

mothers of twins or triplets—require a little extra equipment to make things a little easier. Start with a good pump (you can rent one at the hospital or purchase a new one). There's a good chance your babies might be born a bit early and may be staying in the NICU, so you'll need it to pump and store your breast milk to keep up your supply while you're apart (actually, you'll likely need a pump even if your babies do come home with you, so consider it a good investment). To make the actual act of breastfeeding easier, consider getting a nursing pillow specially designed for twins (look for one with a large, firm surface that can help support two babies at once). If you can't find a twin pillow, you can also use rolled up towels or regular pillows to support your back and elbows. Then of course there are the necessary accoutrements: bottles so your partner can feed your pumped milk (or formula if you're supplementing) and you can get a much-needed break, breast pads to absorb leakage, and lanolin ointment (find it in most drugstores) to soothe sore nipples.

"I'm confused by some things in the bag the nurse just gave me. What are they?"

Every hospital is different in what it sends you home with, but you should get most of these items.

PERIBOTTLE Fill the peribottle with warm water and squirt it on yourself as you go to the bathroom. It's also good for relieving itchiness when you can't scratch.

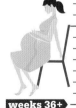

weeks 36+

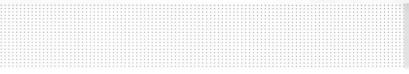
SUPER-THICK PADS You'll still have a very heavy flow after you give birth, so heavy-duty pads are a necessity.

DOUGHNUT PILLOW Sitting down ain't easy in the days following delivery, but this round, open pillow will certainly help.

SKIN NUMBING SPRAY If you have a tear or episiotomy, this will help with the pain.

WITCH HAZEL PADS Whether or not you have hemorrhoids, these will help sooth your entire tender area. Chilling them may provide even more relief.

SITZ BATH This sits over your toilet and allows you to soak your delivery area in warm water, causing more blood to flow there to promote healing.

DISPOSABLE MESH UNDIES They also help keep your heavy-duty pads in place. Some moms love the disposable undies for their convenience.

"PUPPY PADS" These waterproof pads can be placed under you while you sleep, just in case. If you don't need them, use them for your babies' changing table.

acronyms

"I've been hearing a lot of acronyms while hanging around the NICU. what do they mean?"

There are definitely a lot of acronyms in the medical world, but the idea is to make it simple, not confusing. Here are a few of the most common ones and what they mean.

CPAP (Continuous Positive Air Pressure) This is a machine that's used to help babies who have poor respiration. It ensures an adequate oxygen supply reaches the lungs and body.

ECMO (Extracorporeal Membrane Oxygenation) Used for babies whose lungs are failing despite other treatments, ECMO takes over the work of the lungs so they can rest and heal.

NEC (Necrotizing Enterocolitis) This is the most common intestinal condition in newborns. The more premature the babies, the greater the risk for NEC.

PDA (Patent Ductus Arteriosus) This occurs when the blood vessel in the heart that connects the aorta to the pulmonary artery remains open after birth. When this happens, blood can flood the vessels in the lungs, causing respiratory problems.

PVL (Periventricular Leukomalacia) Though there are often no signs of PVL, this type of brain injury is something that doctors look out for in preemies.

RDS (Respiratory Distress Syndrome) The most common condition behind babies who are having trouble breathing, this condition is very treatable.

ROP (Retinopathy of Prematurity) This abnormal growth of the blood vessels in an infant's eye is something to watch out for in very premature babies (especially those weighing less than 3 pounds).

BPD (Bronchopulmonary Dysplasia) This chronic lung condition affects newborn babies who were either put on a breathing machine after birth or were born prematurely.

IVH (Intraventricular Hemorrhage) of the newborn This is when there is bleeding into the fluid-filled areas (ventricles) surrounded by the brain.

NG TUBE OR OG TUBE (Nasogastric Tube or Orogastric Tube) These tubes may be used to feed the babies or give them medicine.

PICC OR PIC LINE (Peripherally Inserted Central Catheter) This special IV line is used to provide fluids into a vein. A PICC line is usually very stable and lasts longer than a typical IV.

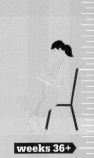

weeks 36+

chapter

now what do I do with these things?

eight

you made it through pregnancy—and delivery. It's over! Actually, of course, it's only just beginning. Now you have to figure out motherhood: the feeding, the bathing, the breast-feeding, the diaper changing, all times two . . . or three . . . or four! Relax, you'll get the hang of everything. Eventually, you'll know what to do for your babies better than anyone in the world. Just don't freak out if adjusting to this new life doesn't "come naturally"—it's a little bit tougher for some than it is for others. These first few weeks are a time for resting, recovering, and getting to know your babes as you and your partner figure out how to navigate life with these amazing new additions to your family!

your to-do list

- Schedule postpartum appointment

- Schedule babies' first checkup

- Track babies' feedings

- Keep up with your Kegels

▶ Check out even more new-mom advice at TheBump.com/newborn

what you're in for…

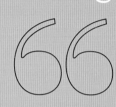

All this blood really freaks me out!

SO CUTE . . . SO LITTLE . . . SO MANY

Everything hurts!

I CAN'T STOP CRYING.

Are you sure I can keep these tiny creatures alive?

I hope my nipples get used to this breastfeeding thing soon.

I'm so overwhelmed!

Engorgement sucks!

PEOPLE KEEP ASKING IF THERE'S ANOTHER BABY IN THERE. YES, I'M STILL HUGE. THANKS.

MAN, PUSHING REALLY BEAT ME UP—I LOOK TERRIBLE!

I am terrified to poop!

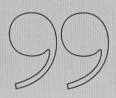

on your mind...

❧ care basics

"When will I need to take my babies to the pediatrician for the first time?"

Most pediatricians will want to see babies at least at birth, 2 to 4 days after birth, and then at 2, 4, 6, 9, and 12 months, the minimum recommended by the American Academy of Pediatrics. Every doctor's preferences are different, though, and some ask to see babies more often. Talk to yours to see what sort of schedule to expect.

"How do I care for the umbilical cord stump?"

The recommendations for this have changed a lot in recent years, and not all doctors agree—so ask your pediatrician what she recommends. Some say to simply keep the cord dry until it falls off and heals on its own (as in, don't put anything on it, including water). We know of others who recommend dabbing it with alcohol during diaper changes to make it dry up and heal faster—in about 2 weeks, as opposed to the month it could take when left alone. Why the rush? The sooner it heals, the sooner you can give babies a bath in the tub. (You'll have to sponge-bathe until then.)

"What the heck am I supposed to do with this penis?"

Take it easy—penises aren't as complicated as they seem. In general, just keep it clean and try to dodge the pee fountains. If your son was circumcised, you'll need to clean the region two or three times a day with warm water (no soap) and apply a lubricant during diaper changes (your pediatrician or hospital should provide one). Also, watch for (rare) signs of infection, like fever, sudden swelling or redness, smelly discharge or pus, or skin that is warm to the touch. (Some of the redness and yellow scabbing is normal and should fade in 7 to 10 days.) After the penis has healed, it's on to basic hygiene. (Clean it with a wipe at diaper changes, and with water in the tub.) If your son still has his foreskin, you don't have to clean under it. (Never try to pull it back before it has separated from the tip of the penis—usually by age 5 or so.) Simply wash on top of it with warm water and gentle soap, the same as you would anywhere else. And don't freak if you see white, pearl-like lumps under the foreskin. These are just the skin cells that are shed when the foreskin separates.

"How do I know my twins are eating enough? What's the recommended amount?"

There's more uncertainty involved if you're feeding straight from the breast instead of a bottle, since you can't exactly see those little milliliter lines. So look for cues from your babies. If you have some satisfied customers, there will be plenty of output in the diapers, and they'll seem more content between feedings. You'll also be seeing your pediatrician on a regular basis, and she'll be able to tell you if they are both gaining enough weight. Babies will typically not consume a lot the first week,

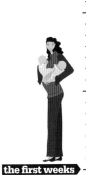

the first weeks

but their volume will increase greatly over time, going from just 10 or 20 milliliters to 60 or more.

"How do you tell their bottles apart?"

Worried about mixing up who's drinking what and how much during each feeding? Place the bottles in the same position the babies are in (so if Suzy is to the left of Sammy, put the bottle on the left side of the table or counter behind her) when you put the bottle down to burp. You can also try marking the outside of the bottle with an initial or symbol. But don't worry too much about exchanging cooties at this point—it's part of life with newborn multiples and bound to happen at some point. At the end of the day, you can sterilize all the bottles by running them through the dishwasher.

"How can I feed them both at the same time?"

Simultaneous dining is highly recommended if you plan on getting any sleep for the next few months, or finding time to do much more than be a feeding and burping machine. It can be challenging at first but will greatly simplify your life once you get the hang of it. There are several methods for coordinating feedings, but with any of them, just remember to take frequent burping breaks.

• Use a twin baby pillow. These large, U-shaped pillows can work for both breast- and bottle-feedings. For breastfeeding, sit in the center with a baby on either side, head out and feet toward your body (known as the classic football hold). Once they're in position, they can both nurse at the same time. You can also prop them up in the twin pillow and use bottles (great for times when your partner is handling the feedings).

• Bed or throw pillows. They're a little more awkward to position, but ordinary pillows can also be arranged to do the trick. For nursing, try propping the pillows under your elbows and holding one baby in front across your lap (a cradle hold) while the other stays in a football hold with his feet facing your body, or have both babies in front of you with their feet crisscrossed. Some parents have also found success with simply propping the babies up, facing you, with their head on the pillow, positioned the long way.

• Bring in the car seat. If you're sticking purely with the bottle, try strapping each baby into her car or infant carrier. Hold a bottle in each hand, and sit cross-legged on the floor in between the carriers.

"I don't know if I'm burping them right. How am I supposed to do it?"

Burping expels air swallowed during feeding and helps eliminate spit-up, crankiness, and gas. Burp when you switch breasts, or after babies drink 2 to 3 ounces. Try these tips:

• Lay one baby belly-down on your lap, with his head above his chest, and pat his back.

"how did the nurses swaddle my babies so perfectly? I suck at this."

First, cut yourself some slack. Those nurses have had a ton of practice! You'll get the hang of it if you keep trying—here are the basic instructions:

STEP 1 Spread out a lightweight blanket in a diamond shape. Picture a clock face.

STEP 2 Fold the top corner (12 o'clock) down about 6 inches. Place baby's head just above the fold, her feet pointing at 6 o'clock.

STEP 3 Take the right corner (3 o'clock), and wrap it over her left arm and chest. Tuck it behind her back, under her right arm.

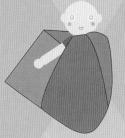

STEP 4 Take the 6 o'clock corner, and pull it up over her feet. Tuck the blanket under her chin.

STEP 5 Pull the final corner (9 o'clock) across her body and around and under her back. Don't be afraid to make it snug.

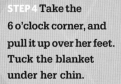

the first weeks

- Hold baby facing your chest, with his chin on your shoulder. Use one hand to support his head and the other to rub or pat his back. Or face him outward and leaning a bit forward, supporting his neck and chest with one hand.
- Once baby can hold his head up, you can hold him against your body, facing outward. Gently apply presure on his stomach as you walk around the room.

"How can I get them on the same schedule?"

Ask almost any parent of multiples whose children are out of infancy, and they'll tell you the secret to maintaining their sanity in those early days was getting those babies on the same schedule. Think of it this way: It can take up to an hour for just one feeding, and newborns have to eat every two to four hours. If you feed them one at a time, you'll be going back-to-back for much of the day (and night). You could probably keep this up for a day or two, but after about a week you'd be a resident of Crazytown.

So, while it seems counterintuitive to wake up a newborn who is sleeping peacefully, the reality is that in order to survive the ensuing chaos that comes with caring for two or more new babies, you need to get them eating and sleeping at approximately the same time. When one baby wakes to eat, it's time to wake the other. Some families are more regimented than others—waking one or both babies to eat exactly every 2 to 3 hours. Others just let one baby take the lead and follow a more approximate schedule. Once they're up, feed them (ideally at the same time), burp them, and do a diaper change. By that point, they (and you!) should probably be ready for another nap.

"What do I need when I'm bringing my babies home from the hospital?"

Most hospitals won't let you go past the exit doors without your babies safely strapped into their infant carriers (aka car seats). Just make sure there is a 4 pounds weight limitation, not 5 pounds. Once you're home, you'll need plenty of diapers, wipes, bottles and nipples, some formula if you're planning to bottle-feed or supplement, and at least one crib for them to sleep in. It's also helpful to have a breast pump, infant washtub, changing table, and diaper pail on hand. The rest of your baby shower booty will come in handy at some point, but probably not immediately.

"Should I set up separate rooms or put them in one?"

In the hazy newborn days, it can make your life much easier if they're sharing the same space, especially when you're stumbling around for those frequent middle-of-the-night feedings. It also helps get them on the same schedule when you're not schlepping from one room to the next. And your tots are likely comforted by each other's presence. There's plenty of time, if you have the space, to give them each their own room as they get bigger (and want some privacy).

checklist

"what are the absolute essentials I need to care for babies?"

You'll get good use out of all the items in your baby health-care kit, whether you choose to buy an all-in-one set or each product individually.

what you need

- **THERMOMETER** Buy a digital rectal thermometer. It's as effective as glass, without risk of breaking. You should rely on core temperature for babies, which means ear and forehead thermometers are out for now. Use petroleum jelly to lubricate the thermometer.

- **NAIL CLIPPERS OR FILE** Babies' nails grow like crazy. Get clippers designed for infants so you don't snip their skin by mistake. If even the miniature clippers seem too scary, stick with filing.

- **BULB SYRINGE** For tiny noses clogged up with mucus, nasal aspirators are the way to go.

- **BABY TYLENOL** If your newborn has a fever, call the pediatrician and pay a visit. Docs generally prefer to see such new babies in person.

- **SALINE** To get dried-up mucus off babies' faces.

- **COTTON SWABS AND BALLS** Moisten these to clean out gooky eyes.

- **AQUAPHOR** This can be used for all kinds of minor irritations, from dry skin and lips to diaper rash.

- **BABY COMB/SOFT-BRISTLE BRUSH** Especially if your infants have hair or cradle cap.

- **GAS DROPS OR GRIPE WATER** Though there's no clinical evidence that these gas remedies work, many parents swear by them. They're benign enough that if they seem to work for you, use them.

- **ANTIBIOTIC CREAMS** Talk to your doctor before using Neosporin or other, similar topical creams.

the first weeks

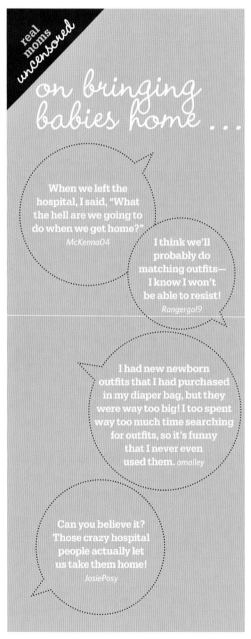

real moms *uncensored*

on bringing babies home . . .

When we left the hospital, I said, "What the hell are we going to do when we get home?"
McKenna04

I think we'll probably do matching outfits— I know I won't be able to resist!
Rangergal9

I had new newborn outfits that I had purchased in my diaper bag, but they were way too big! I too spent way too much time searching for outfits, so it's funny that I never even used them. *omalley*

Can you believe it? Those crazy hospital people actually let us take them home!
JosiePosy

in your head

"I wish someone would take these babies away for a few days while I sleep. Does that make me a bad mother?"

No, it makes you normal. Your exhaustion has no implications for your love for your children, or your maternal abilities. Hang in there—it gets better. In the meantime, ask for help. Have someone (your partner? your mom? a friend?) take over baby duty for an afternoon while you sleep between feedings. Also ask someone to go to the grocery store for you, or to cook. Seriously—take advantage of all the help you can get. You deserve it.

"What does postpartum depression feel like? Do I have it?"

Postpartum depression (aka PPD) is a serious illness that affects as many as 20 percent of new moms, causing extreme sadness or anger in the weeks or months after the babies arrive. Moms of multiples are at an even greater risk for this, as studies show you are 43 percent more likely than a mom of a singleton to be afflicted with PPD. So be vigilant in monitoring your emotions and moods after delivery. Symptoms of PPD include feeling profoundly sad, hopeless, helpless, irritable, or extremely exhausted, and you may find yourself crying, having trouble eating, or forgetting things. You might also be unable to—or just not want to—take care of yourself and/or the babies. Some women feel better in a few weeks, and others suffer for months or a year or longer; in some cases, PPD does not present itself until some time after the babies arrive, so, while

"I'm a wreck about my babies' first bath! what do I need?"

When you're bathing multiples, you want to have your partner or another helper standing by with a towel. Start from the top, one baby in the bath at a time, and move your way down. When you are done with each baby, hand her off to the helper to be dried and dressed.

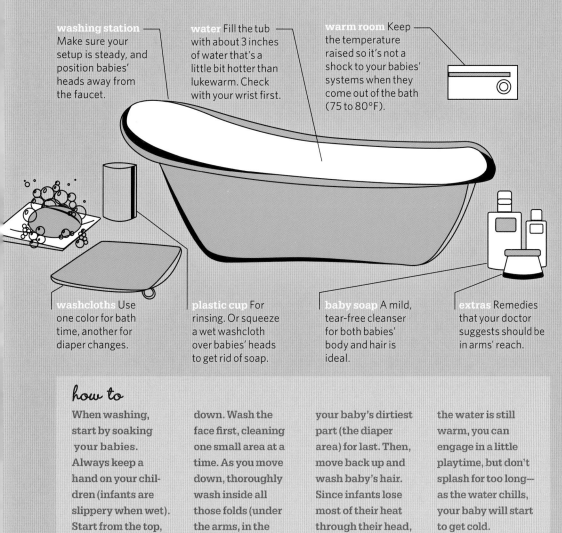

washing station Make sure your setup is steady, and position babies' heads away from the faucet.

water Fill the tub with about 3 inches of water that's a little bit hotter than lukewarm. Check with your wrist first.

warm room Keep the temperature raised so it's not a shock to your babies' systems when they come out of the bath (75 to 80°F).

washcloths Use one color for bath time, another for diaper changes.

plastic cup For rinsing. Or squeeze a wet washcloth over babies' heads to get rid of soap.

baby soap A mild, tear-free cleanser for both babies' body and hair is ideal.

extras Remedies that your doctor suggests should be in arms' reach.

how to

When washing, start by soaking your babies. Always keep a hand on your children (infants are slippery when wet). Start from the top, one baby at a time, and work your way down. Wash the face first, cleaning one small area at a time. As you move down, thoroughly wash inside all those folds (under the arms, in the neck, the genital area, etc.). Save your baby's dirtiest part (the diaper area) for last. Then, move back up and wash baby's hair. Since infants lose most of their heat through their head, this should be your very last move. If the water is still warm, you can engage in a little playtime, but don't splash for too long-- as the water chills, your baby will start to get cold.

the first weeks

you may feel fine when your children are newborns, depression can set in months later. However, keep in mind that if you're feeling down, isolated, and emotionally fragile just after delivery, it doesn't necessarily mean that you have PPD. Lots of moms suffer from something called "baby blues." It's totally normal to feel sad or overwhelmed at first, and to need a good cry now and then. Make sure not to neglect yourself—sleep when you can, eat well, and ask for help when you need it. The baby blues should pass in a few weeks. If they don't or your symptoms get more extreme, talk to your doctor in order to assess whether you have PPD.

If you think you might have PPD, talk to your doctor about treatment options. Luckily, PPD is a treatable form of depression, so get help.

"I still look pregnant. How long will it last?"

Give your body a break—it just went through a heck of a lot of stretching and strain, and it will take time for it to recover. The good news? Your leftover bump should deflate (for the most part) within a few weeks, as your uterus shrinks back down to its regular, plum-size proportions. As for your extra padding, get active as soon as your OB says it's okay, eat right, and you'll start seeing results. Remember, though, that your body went through 9 months of growing and changing. It might take just as long to feel like your old self.

"What happens if I can't tell my twins apart?"

Even though they're twins, your babies will likely have very different personalities, and you'll soon get to know which one is "the quiet one" and which is "the bossy one," or some combination of both. But in the early days, especially with identical twins, you may worry that the baby you've been calling Jake for the past few days was really the one you named Josh at birth. To minimize confusion, take a close look at both babies, because even identicals can have unique features, such as birthmarks or moles. Some parents will paint a toenail for each twin, either using different colors or painting just one. You can also try putting an anklet or different bracelets on one or both babies. When they get older they'll probably try and trick you, but don't worry—you'll know who's who.

"How do I deal when they're all crying at the same time?"

Every mom- (and dad-) to-be has worried about the time when she or he will be alone, surrounded by screaming infants demanding immediate attention. It's a fact that babies cry, sometimes a lot. After all, it's their primary method of communication, and it will occur when they're hungry, wet, overstimulated, gassy, uncomfortable, or just plain tired. Sometimes placing one baby in a carrier and keeping her close to you while holding or soothing the other can stop

newborn care

cleaning the umbilical cord

During diaper changes, wipe around the area with an alcohol wipe (check with your OB; some think it's better to leave it alone). The remaining cord should fall off in a few weeks. Call your doctor if you see redness, warmth, swelling, or if it still hasn't fallen off in 4 to 6 weeks.

trimming long nails

It's important to keep your babies' nails short so they don't scratch their face or eyes. The best way to do this is to trim them with infant-size clippers or file them down while the babies are sleeping. It might be tempting, but skip the scissors—or biting your new-borns' nails.

cleaning out ear wax

Don't stick anything, including Q-tips, into your babies' ear canal, even if you spot wax inside. Eventually, it'll clear out on its own.

bathing

Limit bathing to a few times a week (or as needed). The truth is, infants don't get that dirty (exception: very messy poops or spit-ups). And until your babies' umbilical cords have fallen off, don't immerse their bellies.

changing diapers

Changing them ASAP is the key to fighting rashes. Girl tip: Wipe front to back to avoid urinary tract infections. Boy tip: It's normal for him to get erections during diaper changes.

the screaming and restore calm. But realize there are going to be days when both babies cry, and in most cases it's okay if you're not responding to both immediately. In time, they'll also learn to soothe themselves. And think of it this way: Twins learn to be more resilient early on, since their needs aren't always immediately being met.

"I feel like the crying is contagious. Is it possible for one baby to cry when he hears the other(s)?"
It's possible—after all, laughter can also be contagious, for babies and adults. Or it could just be that one baby is annoyed that his sibling is keeping him up or disturbing his peace.

It can help to put together a support team of friends and family to deal with crying babies and the like, especially when you're feeling sleep deprived and stressed out. You may also want to establish a distress code to signal your partner or another caregiver when you're at your breaking point and need to step away from all the crying.

"Is there anything to the idea that the older twin is usually the bossy one?"
Some moms will swear that their firstborn is the more talkative, outgoing one, but others say the whole birth-order thing—even with twins—is hogwash. And while your twins may share many characteristics (similar hair and eye color, a taste for anything chocolaty),

they're certainly going to grow up to be two separate people. Most parents of multiples say their children develop very different personalities even from an early age. And the more different they are, the more interesting life will be.

is it normal?

"I heard my babies' eyes might change color. When would that happen?"
You heard right. Babies often switch eye color after birth. Some doctors say it takes between 4 and 6 months to see the true hue, but it's possible for them to change later—even after a year. If you are trying to predict the final color, the biggest clue is your own eye color (and your mate's, of course).

"What's up with these first poops?!"
That dark greenish-black, gooey, sticky stuff in their diapers is called meconium, and it's made up of all the stuff your babies were swallowing in utero (amniotic fluid, lanugo, bile, mucus, dead skin cells—yummy).

After a few bowel movements, babies will switch over to mustard-yellow poop if you're breastfeeding. It will probably look as though it has seeds in it, and shouldn't smell very bad (score one for nursing!). Breast milk is digested fast, so the babies might poop after almost every feeding at first. If you are formula feeding, their stool can be yellow, brown, or green, and will smell a little stronger.

See something weird in your babies' diaper? If the poop is hard and pebble-like, red (could

diaper bag

size Consider your needs and whether you'll be carrying a regular bag too. Remember, if there's extra room, you'll fill it.

straps Adjustable straps prevent any slipping. They're also key if more than one person is using the bag.

closure A zipper's ideal for holding everything in. Stay away from Velcro; the ripping noise it makes can wake sleeping babies.

extra pockets Lots of outer pockets make it quick to find a pacifier, bottle, cell phone, or keys.

base A bag that stands up on its own is easier to reach into.

color If you plan to share, choose a color that suits everyone's taste.

changing pad Make sure it's big enough to be useful—especially as your babies grow.

inside the bag

- diapers (2 for every 2 hours, plus a few extra)
- extra changing pad or blanket
- wipes and cream
- important numbers
- extra money
- spare keys
- burp cloths or washcloths (2 per baby)
- pacifiers
- bottles and formula
- extra blanket
- change of clothes
- hats (1 per baby)
- zipper-top bags
- nursing cover

be blood), black (could be digested blood), or white (could signal a liver problem), give the pediatrician a ring. Any other colors are fine.

"Help—my 2-day-olds are losing weight! What should I do?"

You should stop freaking out, pronto. Babies can lose up to 10 percent of their birth weight in the first week of life. We repeat, it's *normal*. As long as your babies are feeding regularly, peeing, and pooping, they're fine. Most make it back up to their birth weight within 2 weeks.

"I am SO tired, I have a black eye, and my chest hurts. What gives?"

Labor is no picnic. Your body just went through a lot, and it's normal to feel (and see) the strain. And strain, actually, is what probably caused your shiner (you were probably "pushing" with your face during delivery), as well as the achy chest (strained chest muscles, also from pushing). The exhaustion, of course, is par for the course, and you're probably sore pretty much all over. Get as much rest as you can, and report all of your symptoms to your nurse or OB, just to be sure everything is peachy.

"Am I supposed to be bleeding this much? When will it stop?"

Bleeding a lot in the days (and weeks) after delivery is normal. What you're seeing isn't only blood. It's called "lochia" and it contains other leftover stuff from inside your uterus, like mucus and tissue. It's likely to be as heavy as your period (remember way back when you had periods?) or even heavier, and

it might gush when you stand, or when you breastfeed. This discharge should go from red to pink in the next three weeks or so, eventually turning brown and then a pale yellow or white. Stock up on pads for these next few weeks, and get medical attention immediately if it becomes smelly or turns bright red again after it turns pink or brown, or if you pass a clot bigger than a golf ball (could signal a hemorrhage).

"Why am I sweating through my PJs?"

No one knows for sure, but it's probably your body getting rid of the extra water you've been carrying. (You'll pee a lot of the excess fluids out as well.) Hormones may play a role too—namely, the drastic drop in estrogen just after you deliver. This should ease up in a few weeks, but it might last a little longer if you're breastfeeding. It might seem counterintuitive, but staying extra hydrated can help. To keep comfy at night, stash a stack of tees bedside.

breastfeeding 411

"I don't think anything is coming out of my boobs when my 2-day-olds suck. Should I give them formula too?"

No, and no. If your babies are sucking regularly (every 2 to 3 hours), they are almost definitely getting your colostrum (even if you can't see it). They need only about a teaspoon worth at each feeding. Rest assured that your milk should come flooding in on about day 3 or 4. Don't stop now—keep your babies breastfeeding regularly to help stimulate your body to fill your boobs. And don't be afraid; your body was made to breastfeed.

"I get cramps when I breastfeed— is that supposed to happen?"

When babies suck, your body makes oxytocin (the same hormone that they use to induce labor). This stuff makes your uterus contract. Why do you need to have contractions now that your babies are out? Well, your uterus grew a heck of a lot during pregnancy, and it's on its way back down. The contractions help it shrink. (You can even feel it shrinking by pressing softly on your tummy.) They can be uncomfortable, but the pains should let up within a week. (If they stick around longer, talk to your OB to make sure there's nothing else going on.)

"My breasts are suddenly enormous and they hurt so badly! What do I do?"

On the bright side, congrats—your milk came in! You're engorged, meaning your body just filled your boobs to bursting (don't worry—they won't really burst). It's no fun (at all), but it won't last forever. In the next 24 to 48 hours, your milk supply should level out, and your breasts will soften up. In the meantime, you can relieve the pain by consistently nursing (not pumping) every 2 to 3 hours, even if you have to wake your babies for the meal. If your boobs are so rock hard that the babies have

> I used the ice packs I got sent home with from the hospital and stuffed them in my bra. I looked funny but hey, it made them feel sooo much better. *mabzie*

a tough time latching on, express (by hand or pump) a little milk first to soften things up. While one of the babies sucks, give your boob a nice massage to help the milk keep flowing, and keep her on one side until it becomes (relatively) soft. Feeding on just one breast per feeding is fine, as long as baby's satisfied. But, lucky for you, you could try feeding one baby on each breast simultaneously. If you're still in pain, try cold packs for a few minutes after feeding, or experiment with the traditional remedy: fresh cabbage leaves. (Rinse them and put them on your boobs.) Whatever you do, don't skip feedings—breastfeeding is a supply-and-demand affair. Not nursing could cause your milk production to take a permanent dip.

"I'm having a really hard time breast-feeding both my newborns. Is it okay to supplement? Should I use any specific type of formula (like one meant just for preemies)?"

Before you start to supplement, see a lacta-tion consultant to confirm you have the positioning right and your newborns are, in fact, sucking correctly. If your babies were born early, they may have dif-ficulty latching on altogether because they may have a less developed suck reflex. The consultant will also weigh your babies before and after you feed them to determine the actual ounces they are taking in. Chances are you're doing

the first weeks

just fine and you and your baby just need a few more days to hit your groove. Do make sure you are drinking enough water because dehydration is one thing that can drastically reduce milk supply.

"What if I'm not breastfeeding? Can I make my milk go away?"

If you don't breastfeed, your body will stop making milk. (That's just how it works.) You'll have to go through the engorgement phase first. It will probably hurt, but it shouldn't last more than a day or two. At this time, some moms swear by doubled-up sports bras and other booby-restricting clothes. Ice packs and pain relievers might help too. Once your breasts have deflated, they might still leak for a few days before drying up.

❚ the new day-to-day

"I'm leaking pee. Can I make it stop?"

Do your Kegels! (See page 88.) Lots of women are a little leaky after childbirth, thanks to the loss of muscle tone in the perineum. Kegels can help build the muscles back up, which can help you learn to "hold it" again.

"Will I ever poop again? Will it hurt like hell when I do?"

Yes, you'll poop. If you just delivered, it's normal to take a day or two (or three) to have a bowel movement, usually due to a combo of weak tummy muscles, soreness, and plain old fear. And, to be honest, it might hurt. But probably not as much as you fear. And you

won't burst your stitches either. Doing your business just might be a little uncomfortable the first time or two, especially if you have hemorrhoids.

To make it easier, eat fiber, drink lots of liquids, take a walk to get your blood flowing . . . and use a stool softener if necessary. Plus, try your darnedest to relax—tension (in your head and in your butt) definitely won't help matters.

"How long will my c-section cut hurt?"

It will take between 4 and 6 weeks for the incision to heal completely. Constipation can compound the pain, so drink lots of fluids, get up and walk when you can, and pack in the fiber (all of these can help you do a number 2). To further manage pain, use good posture, and hold your tummy when you cough, sneeze, or laugh. If breastfeeding bothers the cut, use a support pillow to get your babies off your abdomen. Call your OB if you get a fever over 100.4 degrees, start hurting a lot worse, or have flu-like symptoms or boob pain, or if your incision turns red, swells, or oozes anything (could be an infection).

"How long will I hurt (down there)?"

Your rate of recovery depends on your physical condition in general and how much labor beat you up, but most moms are feeling a whole lot better by 6 weeks postpartum. (Some sooner, some later.) Every day will get a little better, so try to just take it one achy morning at a time. If you had a tear or an episiotomy, speed up healing by keeping your perineum (the tissue between the vagina and rectum) clean and dry. Change sanitary pads every 4 to 6 hours, or whenever you go to the bathroom. Always move from front to back when removing pads or wiping, and wash your hands before and after. These steps prevent bacteria in your stool (yuck!) from entering your vagina. If it hurts to pee or wipe, use a squirt bottle of warm water to spray the area while you go, and pat dry with gauze when you're done. Witch hazel pads can feel heavenly (line your pad with them), as can a numbing spray like Dermoplast (ask your OB first) and even a few ice cubes in the bathtub. Sitz baths (a few inches of warm water in the tub) are also helpful. Try to take one after every bowel movement. And don't forget your Kegels—they'll help tighten muscles, improve circulation, and ultimately reduce the pain. If you have stitches, don't be surprised when pain turns to itching—this is normal as your perineum heals.

"It hurts to sit. I'm too tired to stand."

If it's not practical to lie down all day (don't we all wish it were?), have someone buy you one of those little inflatable doughnut pillows at the nearest drugstore. You'll feel silly, but it'll help because there won't be any pressure.

"When can I have sex again? Not that I'm in the mood . . . just curious!"

Most new moms get the thumbs up from their health-care providers at around 6 weeks postpartum, depending on the condition of their nether regions. (Are you still bleeding? Have the stitches dissolved?) It takes your uterus and cervix time to heal, even if you had a c-section. When you do get back in the sack, take it slow; it will probably be somewhat uncomfortable the first few times, no matter how you delivered. And if you just aren't ready, that's okay too—listen to your body and keep communicating with your mate.

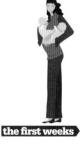

the first weeks

checklist

pregnancy time line

This handy month-by-month pregnancy guide takes you through every stage of the journey, from week 1 to delivery.

weeks 1–8
- Find an OB/GYN
- Schedule prenatal checkup
- Make sure partner has short- and long-term disability
- Figure out how financials will change—you'll have to save money for more than one baby!
- Make a budget
- Have first prenatal checkup (weeks 4–8)
- Eat for three (or more!)

weeks 8–12
- Buy maternity clothes
- Schedule your chorionic villus sampling (weeks 10–14)
- Nuchal translucency screening (weeks 10–12)
- Chromosomal disorder screening (weeks 10–14)
- Visit the doctor
- Hear babies' heartbeats

weeks 12–16
- Start planning maternity leave and postpartum work schedule
- Tell boss and loved ones about pregnancy
- Go to the doctor
- Amniocentesis (weeks 14–16)
- Boost your calories (again!)

weeks 16–20
- Start planning nursery
- Look into child care
- Go to the doctor
- Have midpregnancy ultrasound (weeks 18–20)
- Triple screen aka multiple marker screening or quad screen (weeks 16–18)
- Find out babies' genders
- Feel first baby kicks
- Notice your growing belly
- Register for shower gifts—you'll need two or more of almost everything!

weeks 20–24
- Interview pediatricians
- Research and sign up for childbirth classes
- Visit the doctor

weeks 24–28
- Update or write will, including inheritance and guardianship info
- Purchase life insurance
- Update beneficiaries
- If using doula and child care, start interviews
- Go to the doctor
- Glucose Challenge Screening (weeks 24–28)
- Think about babies' names!

weeks 28–32
- Start fetal kick counts
- Prepare birth plan
- Send thank-you notes
- Freeze postpartum meals
- Start childbirth class
- Have two doctor visits
- Others feel babies move
- Finish painting nursery
- Buy needed baby items
- Pack hospital bag
- Freeze postpartum meals

weeks 32–36
- Assemble first-aid kit
- Prep emergency sheets
- Contact cord blood bank if interested in donating
- Find out about having additional tests
- Have two doctor visits
- Group B strep test (weeks 35–37)
- Have your baby shower
- Start babyproofing home
- Get biophysical profile

weeks 36–delivery
- Visit doctor weekly
- Have nonstress test
- Get car seats inspected

checklist

budget for babies

Here's a list of major purchases and investments over the first year—estimate how much you'll fork over to get a rough answer. And remember . . . the amount you plan to spend doesn't always match the amount you actually do.

one-time expenses:

- Nursery decorating/ remodeling: _____
- Cribs: _____
- Crib mattresses: _____
- Bedding and accessories: _____
- Dresser(s): _____
- Rocking chair: _____
- Changing table: _____
- Baby monitor: _____
- Playpen, bouncy chair(s), or walker(s): _____
- Safety gates: _____
- Baby bathtub(s): _____
- High chairs: _____
- Bottles: _____
- Pump: _____
- Nursing clothes: _____
- Medicine kit: _____
- Stroller: _____
- Baby carrier/sling: _____
- Car seats: _____
- Diaper bag: _____
- Maternity leave salary loss: _____
- Writing/rewriting will: _____

monthly expenses:

- Diapers: _____
- Formula and food: _____
- Clothes: _____
- Toys: _____
- Photo paper and printing: _____
- Extra laundry costs (water, electricity, detergent): _____
- Child care: _____
- Life insurance for you and your partner: _____
- Medical insurance: _____
- Disability insurance: _____
- Medical bills (uncovered and co-pays): _____
- College/education savings: _____
- Contribution to savings: _____

checklist

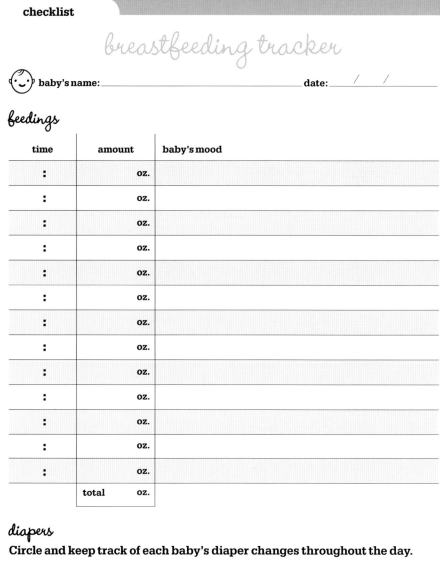

breastfeeding tracker

baby's name: _____   date: ____ / ____ / ____

feedings

time	amount	baby's mood
:	oz.	
:	oz.	
:	oz.	
:	oz.	
:	oz.	
:	oz.	
:	oz.	
:	oz.	
:	oz.	
:	oz.	
:	oz.	
:	oz.	
:	oz.	
	total oz.	

diapers

Circle and keep track of each baby's diaper changes throughout the day.

pee

poo

time   :   :   :   :   :   :   :   :   :   :

checklist

bottle-feeding tracker

baby's name: _____   date: ___/___/___

feedings

time	amount	baby's mood
:	oz.	
:	oz.	
:	oz.	
:	oz.	
:	oz.	
:	oz.	
:	oz.	
:	oz.	
:	oz.	
:	oz.	
:	oz.	
:	oz.	
:	oz.	
total	oz.	

diapers

Circle and keep track of each baby's diaper changes throughout the day.

pee

poo

time   :   :   :   :   :   :   :   :   :   :

checklist

sleep tracker

**Monitor each baby's zzzs. Fill in the date and then
shade in the boxes for hours spent snoozing.**

month: _____

date	time	12 A.M.	2 A.M.	4 A.M.	6 A.M.	8 A.M.	10 A.M.	12 P.M.	2 P.M.	4 P.M.	6 P.M.	8 P.M.	10 P.M.	12 A.M.
	1 ___													
	2 ___													
	3 ___													
	4 ___													
	5 ___													
	6 ___													
	7 ___													
	8 ___													
	9 ___													
	10 ___													
	11 ___													
	12 ___													
	13 ___													
	14 ___													
	15 ___													
	16 ___													
	17 ___													
	18 ___													
	19 ___													
	20 ___													
	21 ___													
	22 ___													
	23 ___													
	24 ___													
	25 ___													
	26 ___													
	27 ___													
	28 ___													
	29 ___													
	30 ___													
	31 ___													

checklist

day-by-day schedule

Keeping track of just one is tricky! Use this guide to stay on top of your multiples' needs.

baby's name: _____ **date:** _____

circle: Mon Tue Wed Thur Fri Sat Sun

time	nursed	diaper	change	medicine
☐ a.m. ☐ p.m.				
☐ a.m. ☐ p.m.				
☐ a.m. ☐ p.m.				
☐ a.m. ☐ p.m.				
☐ a.m. ☐ p.m.				
☐ a.m. ☐ p.m.				
☐ a.m. ☐ p.m.				
☐ a.m. ☐ p.m.				
☐ a.m. ☐ p.m.				
☐ a.m. ☐ p.m.				
☐ a.m. ☐ p.m.				
☐ a.m. ☐ p.m.				
☐ a.m. ☐ p.m.				

notes: _____
_____
_____
_____

baby's name: _____ **date:** _____

circle: Mon Tue Wed Thur Fri Sat Sun

time	nursed	diaper	change	medicine
☐ a.m. ☐ p.m.				
☐ a.m. ☐ p.m.				
☐ a.m. ☐ p.m.				
☐ a.m. ☐ p.m.				
☐ a.m. ☐ p.m.				
☐ a.m. ☐ p.m.				
☐ a.m. ☐ p.m.				
☐ a.m. ☐ p.m.				
☐ a.m. ☐ p.m.				
☐ a.m. ☐ p.m.				
☐ a.m. ☐ p.m.				
☐ a.m. ☐ p.m.				
☐ a.m. ☐ p.m.				

notes: _____
_____
_____
_____

need more advice?

American Academy of Pediatrics
Information on physical, mental, and social health from the nation's leading child health experts. **AAP.org**

American College of Nurse-Midwives
Looking for a midwife? Type in your home address and search the national database for a CNM in your area. ACNM.org

American College of Obstetrics and Gynecologists (ACOG)
A good place to read up-to-date articles on issues affecting women's health. **ACOG.org**

American Pregnancy Association
In addition to being a strong advocacy group, APA also offers forums and educational articles on sexual health, and will help you find a local health professional. **AmericanPregnancy Association.com**

Association of Women's Health, Obstetric and Neonatal Nurses (AWHONN)
Includes articles from government agencies, such as the FDA, CDC, and NIH, that deal with the latest pregnancy-related issues. AWHONN.org

Breastfeeding.com
Answers to all of your breastfeeding questions, plus a supportive breast-feeding community. **Breastfeeding.com**

La Leche League International
Connect with moms in your area and get helpful breastfeeding tips from experienced lactation consultants. LLLI.org

Lamaze International
A nonprofit organization that promotes a natural, healthy, and safe approach to pregnancy, childbirth, and early parenting. **Lamaze.org**

March of Dimes
Dedicated to improving the health of babies by preventing birth defects, premature birth, and infant mortality. MoDimes.org

National Center for Fathering
A great resource for dads and dads-to-be looking for advice and more information on their rights as fathers. Fathers.com

National Women's Health Resource Center
Features recent health reports, nutritional guides, and a pregnancy and parenting center. **HealthyWomen.org**

National Institute of Child Health and Human Development
Conducts studies on health. Find out about a conference or event that the NICHD may be holding in your area. NICHD.NIH.gov

National Organization of Mothers of Twins Clubs
Get connected with other moms in your area who also have twins. NOMOTC.org

National Organization of Single Mothers
Focused on helping single mothers cope with everyday challenges. SingleMothers.org

United States Department of Labor
Information and key news about the Family and Medical Leave Act. DOL.gov/whd/fmla/index.htm

_____

TheBump.com
The most active mommy community on the Web, with the inside scoop on fertility, pregnancy, birth, and everything baby through stage-by-stage advice, interactive tools, and real birth stories.

---

talk to other moms and dads of multiples 24/7 on TheBump.com/multiples

mom-to-be lingo from TheBump.com/boards

BBT Basal Body Temperature
BC Birth Control
BD Baby Dance (baby-making sex)
BF or BF'ing Breastfeeding
BFP Big Fat Positive (home pregnancy test result)

BW Birth Weight
DH Dear Husband
IB Implantation Bleeding
MS Morning Sickness
OWT Old Wives' Tale

PCOS, PCOD Polycystic Ovary Syndrome/Disease
PIT Pitocin
SAHM Stay-at-home mom
US or u/s Ultrasound
VBAC Vaginal Birth after Cesarian

index

a

b

c

acknowledgments

Congrats, you made it through the whole nine months and beyond. I want to give a great big thanks to all the people who helped create this book:

The million-plus moms on TheBump.com for asking and answering just about every question there is.

Erin Van Vuuren and Paula Kashtan for probing into the wonder of pregnancy and babies to find out every tip, trick, or trend for each month; and Maya Cohen and Alyssa Schaffer for their reporting and insights on twins, triplets, and beyond.

The Bump team: Rebecca Dolgin, Brooke Alovis, and Kelly Crook for not even flinching over varicose veins (in the vulva no less), vaginal tears , or the details of versioning.

My good friend and agent, Chris Tomasino.

My husband, cofounder, and partner, David Liu, and my own babies, Havana, Cairo, and Dublin.

credits

experts

Shoshana Bennett, PhD
Author of *Postpartum Depression for Dummies*

Denise Gershwin, CNM
Certified Nurse-Midwife

**Melissa Gould;
Ellie Miller**
Founding Partners of Ellie & Melissa, The Baby Planners

Kathleen A. Hale, BSN, RN, MS, NE-BC
Associate VP of Nursing at Maine Medical Center

**Corky Harvey,
MS, RN, IBCLC;
Wendy Haldeman,
MS, RN, IBCLC**
Cofounders and Co-owners of The Pump Station & Nurtury

Conner Herman; Kira Ryan
Cofounders of Dream Team Baby

Maria Kammerer, CNM
Certified Nurse-Midwife

Erika Lenkert
Author of *The Real Deal Guide to Pregnancy*

Jennifer Loomis
Fine-Art Maternity and Family Photographer

Tracy Mallet
Fitness Lifestyle Expert, Author of *Super Fit Mama*

Dr. Vicki Papadeas
Pediatrician at La Guardia Place Pediatrics, NYC

Dr. Paula Prezioso
Pediatrician at Pediatric Associates of New York City

Dr. Ashley Roman
Clinical Assistant Professor of Obstetrics and Gynecology at New York University School of Medicine

Sebastiaan Selders
Senior Product Manager at Britax

Andi Silverman
Author of *Mama Knows Breast: A Beginner's Guide to Breastfeeding*

**Diane Truong, MD, FAAP;
JJ Levenstein, MD, FAAP**
Cofounders of MDMoms

**Dr. Georgia F.
Wortham III, MD**
Obstetrician at Memphis OB/GYN

Maurice L. Druzin, MD,
Chief of Maternal-Fetal Medicine at Lucile Packard Children's Hospital at Stanford University Medical Center

Katherine Economy, MD, MPH
Maternal Fetal Medicine specialist, Brigham and Women's Hospital, Boston, MA

Shelly Vaziri Flais, MD, FAAP
Pediatrician and Author of *Raising Twins, From Pregnancy to Preschool—Advice from a Pediatrician Mom of Twins*

Elizabeth Lyons
Designer and Author, *Ready or Not...Here We Come!*, ElizabethLyons.com

Michael Yaker, MD, FAAP
Westside Pediatrics, New York City

American Academy of Pediatrics

American College of Obstetrics and Gynecology

American Society for Reproductive Medicine

Society for Maternal-Fetal Medicine

William M. Gilbert, MD
Regional Medical Director for Women's Services at Sutter Health, Sacramento, CA

Julie Redfern
Manager of Nutrition Consulting Services at Brigham and Women's Hospital, Boston, MA

moms

Jennifer Beldon, Kristen Case, Jeanine Edwards, Lauren Flanagan, Heather Fleming, Judy Galani-Plasse, Allison Holt, Monica Locksmoe, Julia Lyson, Kari Merkel, Nicole Ragains, Lori Richmond, Alison Salat Bernstein, Lisa Shapiro Dotson, Laura Soloff, Nicole Wertzler

illustrations

LULU*/CWC International, Inc., Megan Rojas, Brown Bird Design, Pig Pen Studio

photography

Sonograms courtesy of GE HealthCare; p. 15, 51, 63, 77, 93, 107, 119: Shutterstock; p. 21: Ragnar Schmuck/Getty Images; p. 25, from top: Meike Bergmann/Jupiter Images, Klaus Arras/StockFood, Istock Photo, Veer, Rita Maas/FoodPix/Getty Images, StockFood/Steven Morris Photography, Veer, Food Collection/StockFood; p. 28: Photo Op/StockFood; p. 31, clockwise from top left: Lew Robertson/Corbis, FoodCollection/StockFood (3), Judd Pilossof/StockFood, Shutterstock, FoodCollection/StockFood; p. 34, 81: Davies+Starr; p. 41: Gazimal/Stone/ Getty Images; p. 59: from top, left to right: Sugar Stock Ltd/Alamy, Stockbyte/Getty Images, Dorling Kindersley/Getty Images, Veronique Leplat/Stockfood Creative/Getty Images, Zabert/Stockfood, Lannretonne/Stockfood, Douglas Johns/Stockfood Creative/Getty Images, Klaus Arras/Stockfood, Laurie Vogt Photography Inc./Stockfood, Crystal Cartier/StockFood Creative/Getty Images, Veer (2), Nicholas Eveleigh/Iconica/Getty Images; p. 69: Mark Lund; p. 85: Getty Images; p. 111: Devon Jarvis; p. 114: Ellen Silverman p. 115: Deborah Jaffe; p. 135: Benjamin Cotton Photographic, Westchester Medical Center; p. 157: Veer.